CW00349755

# Menopause

Dr Rebecca Fox-Spencer

Dr Pam Brown

Menopause
First published – April 2006

**Published by**
**CSF Medical Communications Ltd**
1 Bankside, Lodge Road, Long Hanborough
Oxfordshire, OX29 8LJ, UK
T +44 (0)1993 885370 F +44 (0)1993 881868
*enquiries@bestmedicine.com*
*www.bestmedicine.com*

We are always interested in hearing from anyone
who has anything to add to our Simple Guides.
Please send your comments to *editor@csfmedical.com*.

**Author** Dr Rebecca Fox-Spencer
**Managing Editor** Dr Eleanor Bull
**Medical Editor** Dr Pam Brown
**Science Editor** Dr Scott Chambers
**Production Editor** Emma Catherall
**Layout** Jamie McCansh and Julie Smith
**Operations Manager** Julia Savory
**Publisher** Stephen I'Anson

© CSF Medical Communications Ltd 2006

All rights reserved

ISBN-10: 1-905466-13-7
ISBN-13: 978-190546-613-9

The contents of this *Simple Guide* should not be treated as a substitute for
the medical advice of your own doctor or any other healthcare professional.
You are strongly urged to consult your doctor before taking, stopping or
changing any of the products or lifestyle recommendations referred to in this
book or any other medication that has been prescribed or recommended by
your doctor. Whilst every effort has been made to ensure the accuracy of the
information at the date of publication, CSF Medical Communications Ltd and
The Patients Association accept no responsibility for any errors or omissions or
for any consequences arising from anything included in or excluded from this
*Simple Guide* nor for the contents of any external internet site or other
information source listed and do not endorse any commercial products or
services mentioned.

Printed in Italy.

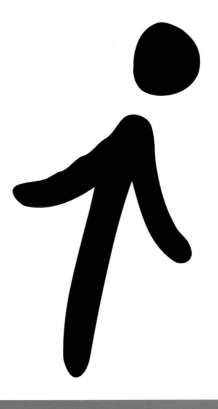

## FOREWORD

### TRISHA MACNAIR
*Doctor and BBC Health Journalist*

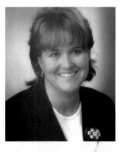 Getting involved in managing your own medical condition – or helping those you love or care for to manage theirs – is a vital step towards keeping as healthy as possible. Whilst doctors, nurses and the rest of your healthcare team can help you with expert advice and guidance, nobody knows your body, your symptoms and what is right for *you* as well as you do.

There is no long-term (chronic) medical condition or illness that I can think of where the person concerned has absolutely no influence at all on their situation. The way you choose to live your life, from the food you eat to the exercise you take, will impact upon your disease, your well-being and how able you are to cope. You are in charge!

Being involved in making choices about your treatment helps you to feel in control of your problems, and makes sure you get the help that you really need. Research clearly shows that when people living with a chronic illness take an active role in looking after themselves, they can bring about significant improvements in their illness and vastly improve the quality of life they enjoy.

Of course, there may be occasions when you feel particularly unwell and it all seems out of your control. Yet most of the time there are plenty of things that you can do in order to reduce the negative effects that your condition can have on your life. This way you feel as good as possible and may even be able to alter the course of your condition.

So how do you gain the confidence and skills to take an active part in managing your condition, communicate with health professionals and work through sometimes worrying and emotive issues? The answer is to become better informed. Reading about your problem, talking to others who have been through similar experiences and hearing what the experts have to say will all help to build up your understanding and help you to take an active role in your own health care.

*Simple Guides* provide an invaluable source of help, giving you the facts that you need in order to understand the key issues and discuss them with your doctors and other professionals involved in your care. The information is presented in an accessible way but without neglecting the important details. Produced independently and under the guidance of medical experts *Menopause* is an evidence-based, balanced and up-to-date review that I hope you will find enables you to play an active part in the successful management of your condition.

# What happens before the menopause?

# WHAT HAPPENS BEFORE THE MENOPAUSE?

Ironically, it may not be until you start to think about the menopause and its effects that you start to learn how your menstrual cycle has been working for all these years.

### THE MENSTRUAL CYCLE

The menstrual cycle is a series of changes in the female reproductive system that occur every 28 days, though the length of the cycle can vary by up to a week in different women. Each cycle begins with up to a week of bleeding from the uterus, known as a menstrual period. You will have started having periods, or menstruating, during puberty (at a point known as the menarche) and it is quite likely that you will continue to menstruate into your late 40s or beyond. During that time, a number of factors can cause temporary breaks in your menstrual cycle, and therefore your periods, including becoming pregnant.

When a girl is born, there are hundreds of thousands of eggs in her ovaries. When she starts her menstrual cycle at puberty, she will lose one of these eggs (an ovum) in each menstrual period, providing she does not become pregnant.

On average, girls start their periods (the menarche) at about 12–13 years old.

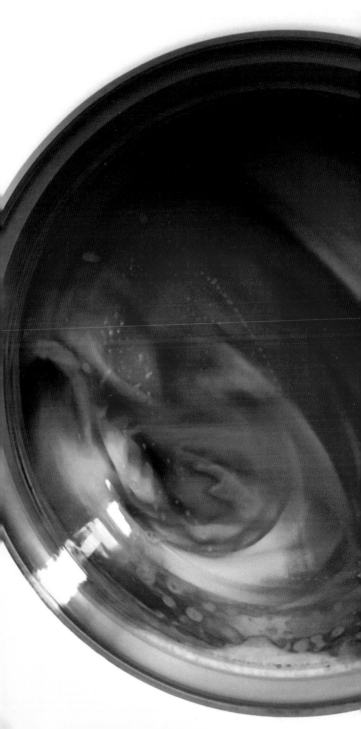

On average, a woman might have around 500 periods in her lifetime, and therefore a large proportion of the original eggs in her ovaries are never shed or fertilised.

The exact timings of the stages of a menstrual cycle vary between different women, but typically during an average 28-day cycle the following events occur:

- **days 1–5** – menstrual bleeding (period)

- **day 7** – eggs in the ovaries begin to 'ripen'

- **day 7–11** – the lining of the uterus starts to thicken, in preparation for the fertilised egg (an egg that has been penetrated by a sperm) to become embedded within its spongy tissue

- **day 14** – the egg is released from the ovary into the fallopian tube, a process known as ovulation

- **day 14–28** – the egg travels down to the uterus. If the egg is fertilised it can implant into the uterus lining, and a pregnancy begins. If it is not fertilised, the egg is released, along with much of the uterus lining, in a period beginning on day 1 of the next cycle.

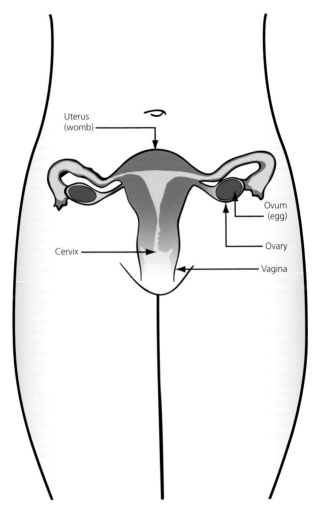

**THE FEMALE REPRODUCTIVE SYSTEM.**

## HORMONES AND THE MENSTRUAL CYCLE

The menstrual cycle is a very complicated process, and yet for some women, their periods are completely predictable and as regular as clockwork. How are these changes, which are so vital for a woman's fertility, controlled so tightly? The most important way in which the menstrual cycle is controlled is by means of your hormones.

There are four main hormones involved in controlling your menstrual cycle.

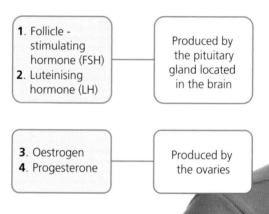

1. Follicle - stimulating hormone (FSH)
2. Luteinising hormone (LH)

Produced by the pituitary gland located in the brain

3. Oestrogen
4. Progesterone

Produced by the ovaries

A hormone is a naturally occurring chemical which is made by specialised cells and released into the blood. The blood carries the hormone to cells elsewhere in the body, where it exerts its effects.

6

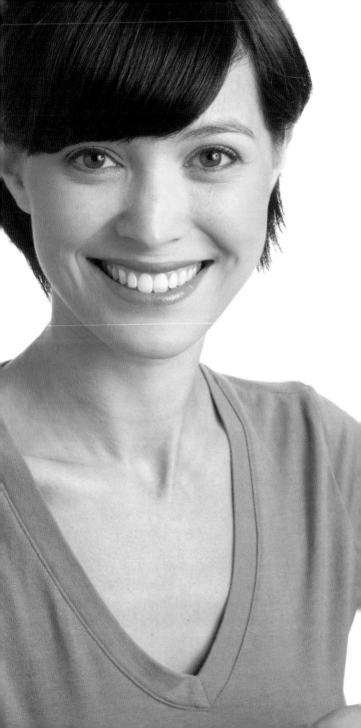

- Early in the cycle, moderate levels of FSH provide a signal for eggs to mature in the ovaries. The eggs are contained in little sacs called follicles. Usually one follicle matures quicker than the rest. FSH also stimulates the ovaries to produce oestrogen.

- Oestrogen encourages the maturing follicle to develop further, and ensures that the lining of the uterus becomes thicker, in preparation for a fertilised egg to be implanted.

- A surge in LH stimulates the process of ovulation, where the mature egg is released from the follicle in the ovary into the fallopian tube.

- The empty follicle turns yellow (called a corpus luteum) and starts producing progesterone. Progesterone causes the lining of the uterus to thicken even more, in preparation for the fertilised egg (known as an embryo) to implant within it.

- The muscles in the walls of the fallopian tube contract gently to propel the egg along. About 6 days after an egg has been released from the ovary, it will reach the uterus. If the egg was fertilised by a sperm whilst in the fallopian tube, then the embryo will implant into the lining of the uterus and levels of progesterone will remain high. This heralds the beginning of pregnancy.

- If the egg was not fertilised, levels of both oestrogen and progesterone fall. This causes the thick lining of the uterus, as well as the unfertilised egg, to be shed during a period.

- The whole process starts again.

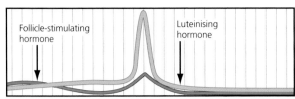

Changes in the hormones released from the brain.

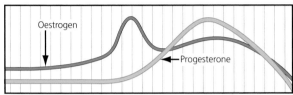

Changes in the hormones released from the ovaries.

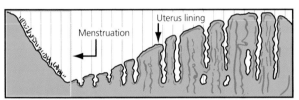

Changes in the thickness and 'sponginess' of the uterus lining.

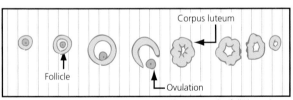

Changes to the follicle and egg.

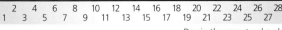

Day in the menstrual cycle.

**CHANGES IN HORMONE LEVELS DURING
THE MENSTRUAL CYCLE.**

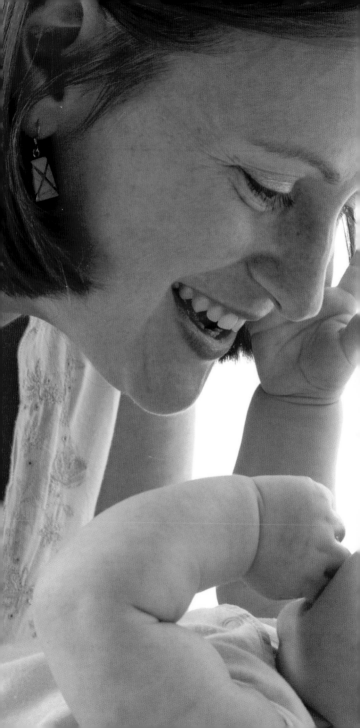

## BREAKS IN MENSTRUATION

There are a number of reasons that you might experience a break between your periods that is longer than normal. Pregnancy is the most obvious of these reasons. Menstrual cycles stop during pregnancy – no new eggs are released and the lining of the uterus must remain thick to support the development of the foetus (developing baby). The menstrual cycle, along with periods, resumes when the baby is born. Breast-feeding, however, affects hormone levels too, and this may delay the menstrual cycle from starting up normally.

Periods may also become irregular or stop for a while for other reasons, such as if you are particularly over- or underweight, emotionally stressed or exercise excessively. In most of these cases, periods will resume again once the problem is addressed. Rarely, a woman may never have any periods at all. This is usually due to problems with the uterus, ovaries or hormone levels. In all women, however, the menstrual cycle stops for good at some point, and this is known as the menopause.

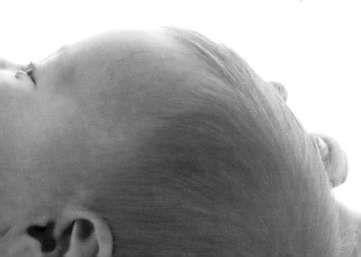

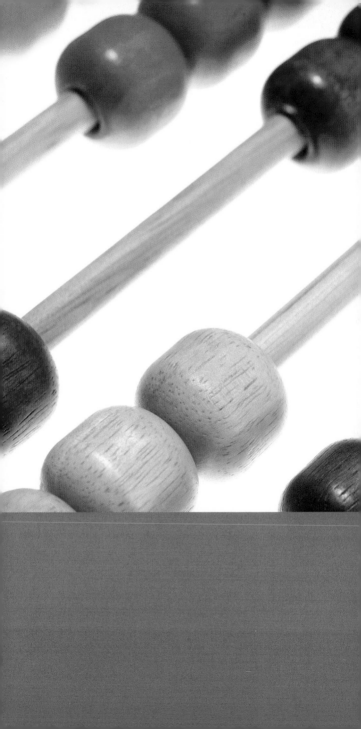

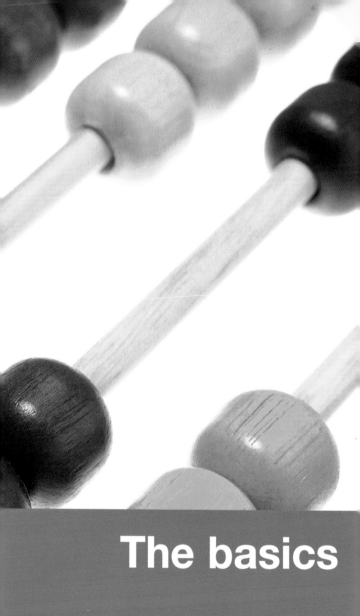

# The basics

# MENOPAUSE – THE BASICS

Recognising the menopause is not as easy as you might think. However, identifying the menopause or 'change of life' is key to the effective management of menopausal symptoms and the avoidance of potential complications.

### WHAT IS THE MENOPAUSE?

You might think that it is obvious, but do you actually know what the menopause is? The simplest definition of the menopause is the last menstrual period you ever experience. This occurs when the levels of the hormones controlling the menstrual cycle have fallen so low that it can no longer happen. It can be difficult to recognise exactly when the menopause occurs because periods can become irregular as you get older.

The generally accepted view is that you can only claim to have had your last period when it occurred at least 1 year previously, and that you have not been pregnant within that year. Experts tend to agree that if you are not yet 50, you should wait for at least 2 years before concluding that you have had your last period.

Confusingly, when people refer to 'the menopause', they are often talking about the gradual changes and symptoms that occur during the few years before and after the last menstrual period. The more accurate name for the period of transition from reproductive to non-reproductive life is the **climacteric phase**.

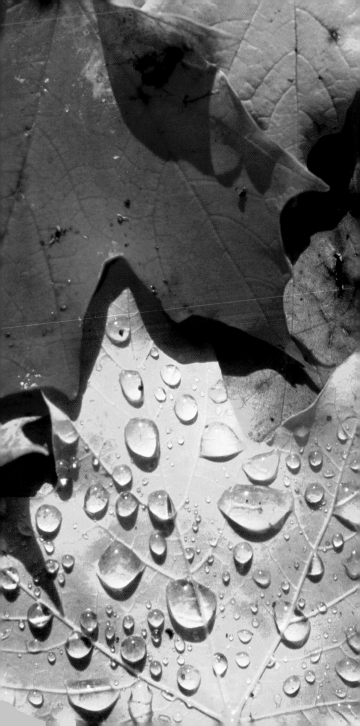

**IMPORTANT DEFINITIONS**

■ **Premenopause** – the entire period of time during which a woman can become pregnant, from puberty to the menopause.

■ **Perimenopause** – this stage usually lasts around 4–5 years, and begins before the menopause itself, at the time when you might first experience menopausal symptoms (e.g. hot flushes, night sweats). Menstrual periods usually become less predictable during this phase. You may notice that they become less or more frequent, less regular, heavier or lighter. When you have had a whole year (or two if you are under 50) without menstrual periods, this marks the end of the perimenopause and the onset of the menopause.

■ **Postmenopause** – the time beyond the last period.

It is important to recognise that whilst the menopause can cause distressing symptoms, it is not strictly an illness. It will happen to every woman who reaches menopausal age. The average age for a woman to reach menopause is 51, though having your last period at any time between the ages of 45 and 55 is considered completely normal.

When we refer to 'menopausal symptoms', we specifically mean symptoms that occur any time during the climacteric phase.

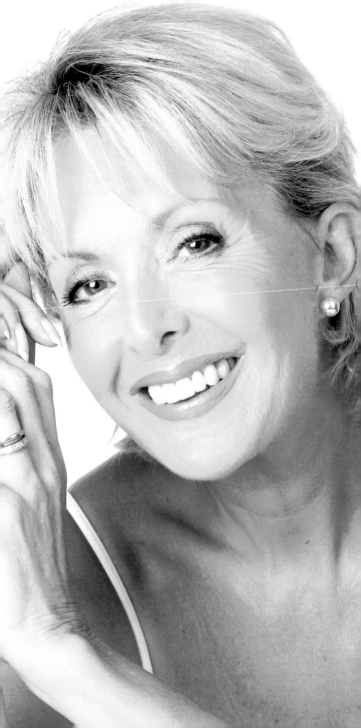

## WHY DOES IT HAPPEN?

Your menstrual cycle is controlled by two
hormones that are produced in the pituitary gland
in the brain (FSH and LH) and two that are
generated in the ovaries (oestrogen and
progesterone). As you approach the menopause,
FSH and LH continue to be produced by the
pituitary gland as normal. However, as your
ovaries get older they no longer respond to FSH
and LH as they should and, as a result, less and
less oestrogen and progesterone is produced.
The menopause occurs at the point at which
the ovaries no longer produce enough of these
hormones to sustain the menstrual cycle.

In summary, when you go through the
menopause, your oestrogen and progesterone
levels fall dramatically as the ovaries stop
responding to FSH and LH produced by
the pituitary gland in the brain. In
an attempt to get your ovaries
to do their job properly,
the brain actually starts
churning out more
FSH and LH to try

THE PITUITARY, A PEA-SHAPED GLAND HANGING FROM THE
BASE OF THE BRAIN, PRODUCES THE HORMONES THAT
CONTROL THE MENSTRUAL CYCLE.

and get the message across! This doesn't work; your ovaries cannot be convinced to come out of retirement! However, the brain's persistence to produce more and more FSH does have one advantage: high levels of FSH can be detected in the blood or urine and used as a crude test to detect the menopause.

## IDENTIFYING THE MENOPAUSE

The defining feature of the menopause is the stopping of menstrual periods. However, as we have seen, it can be difficult to determine whether you have experienced your final period as they may become infrequent as you approach the menopause. The other reason that you might suspect that you are menopausal is if you experience menopausal symptoms. Only about three-quarters of menopausal women will have symptoms. The more common ones are outlined below.

- Physical symptoms:
    - hot flushes (of your face, neck and chest which last for a few minutes; you may also feel faint, weak or sick)
    - night sweats
    - palpitations (racing/pounding heartbeat)
    - difficulty sleeping
    - headache
    - needing to urinate more often
    - discomfort during urination
    - incontinence.

- Psychological symptoms:
    - irritability
    - depression
    - anxiety
    - mood swings
    - forgetfulness
    - difficulty concentrating.

- Sexual symptoms:
    - dryness in the vagina, leading to discomfort during sex
    - reduced sex drive (libido).

Although such symptoms may help you and your doctor identify when you are approaching the menopause, they are easily mistaken for other conditions and are not particularly useful for pinpointing exactly when the menopause occurs. You can experience symptoms, which may be intermittent, for several years, both before and after the time of your last period.

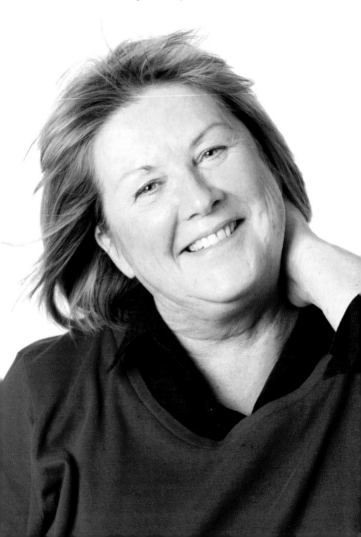

## COMPLICATIONS OF THE MENOPAUSE

Many women sail through the menopause without the need for any medical advice or treatment for symptom relief. However, the changing hormone levels (particularly oestrogen) that characterise the menopause can lead to a number of complications later in life. The complications associated with the menopause are shown below.

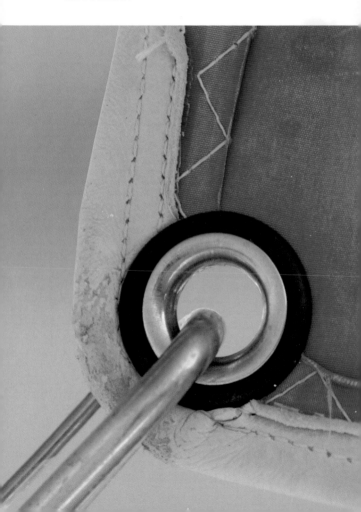

- **Osteoporosis** – a 'bone thinning' disease that makes you susceptible to painful and potentially dangerous fractures.

- **Urogenital problems** – you may start to experience sexual problems, incontinence and urinary tract infections during the perimenopausal phase, but unlike most other menopausal symptoms, these may become more long-term health problems after the onset of the menopause and therefore need to be managed.

- **Cardiovascular disease** – this encompasses a range of problems with the heart and the system of blood vessels that transports blood around the body. It includes problems such as angina, heart attacks and stroke. You are also more likely to suffer from high cholesterol levels after the menopause and the build-up of LDL cholesterol (known as 'bad' cholesterol) can narrow and clog your arteries and thereby increase your risk of cardiovascular disease.

For more information see
**Osteoporosis**

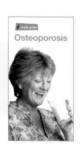

■ **Obesity** – going through the menopause alters the way in which your body stores fat. Prior to the menopause, women generally store excess fat around the hips and thighs, leading to a so-called 'pear-shaped' figure. However, after the menopause, more fat becomes stored around the waist and abdomen, leading to an 'apple-shaped' figure. This body shape is associated with an increased risk of heart disease, type 2 diabetes and certain cancers (e.g. breast cancer).

■ **Dementia** – the links between the menopause and memory problems are not entirely clear, but it appears that female hormones play some role in normal brain function. Although dementia doesn't normally affect women until they are postmenopausal, the onset of the menopause may have a role in the deterioration of memory.

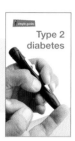

For more information see
**Type 2 diabetes**

Of course, not all menopausal women experience
these complications, but if you know that you are
particularly at risk of any of these conditions,
because of your family history or other pre-
existing medical conditions, you should go
and see your doctor. If your doctor
considers you to be at increased risk, he
or she will advise you on changes
that you should make to your
lifestyle or prescribe you
treatments to try and
prevent these
complications
from occurring.

## HINTS FOR DEALING WITH HOT FLUSHES

■ Wear thin layers of clothing that you can easily remove and put back on again when your temperature fluctuates.

■ Try to avoid hot, spicy foods, caffeinated drinks and alcohol, as these may bring on hot flushes and sweating.

■ Carry tissues with you to wipe your face and body when you sweat.

■ Try to choose cotton nightwear and bedclothes as they are cooler and more breathable than other fabrics.

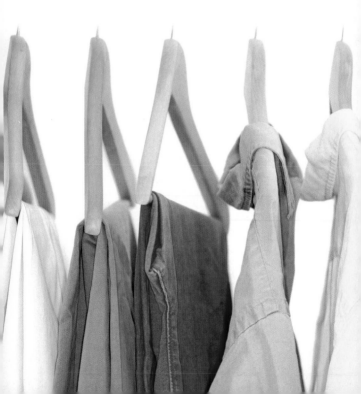

## AIMS OF TREATMENT

Not every woman going through the menopause
will need treatment. In general, there are two
main reasons why your doctor might believe that
you would benefit from taking medication.

1.  If you are suffering moderate or severe
    discomfort from menopausal symptoms. These
    symptoms generally resolve on their own given
    time, but short-term treatment (i.e. treatment
    to reduce the impact of hot flushes) can help
    to alleviate them during this time.
2.  If you are thought to be at risk of
    complications such as osteoporosis, due to a
    family history or previous health problems, for
    example, or because of an early menopause.

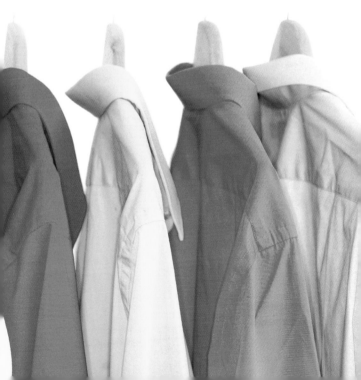

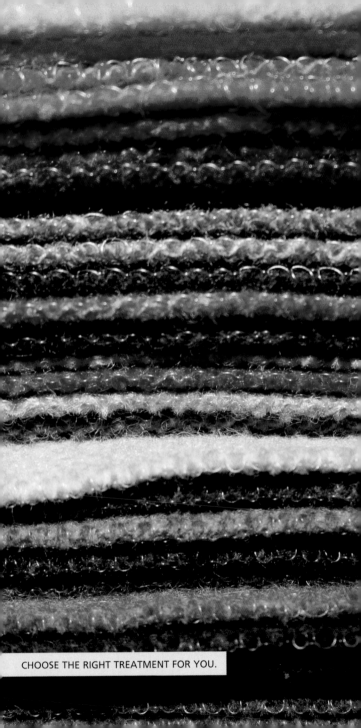

CHOOSE THE RIGHT TREATMENT FOR YOU.

**TREATING THE MENOPAUSE**

The most commonly used treatment for relieving the symptoms of menopause and reducing the risk of future health problems is hormone replacement therapy (HRT). However, as you may have heard in the news, there are some risks associated with using HRT, particularly if it is used for long periods of time.

**POTENTIAL EFFECTS OF LONG-TERM TREATMENT WITH HRT**

| Slight increase in risk | Slight decrease in risk |
| --- | --- |
| Breast cancer | Colorectal cancer |
| Clotting problems (e.g. stroke) | Osteoporosis and fractures |
| Coronary heart disease | |

There are numerous additional treatments and strategies aimed at relieving menopausal symptoms and reducing the risk of future complications. Some drugs, whose effectiveness has been proven in clinical trials, might be prescribed by your doctor. On the other hand, there are various foods and forms of exercise which are believed by many people to be beneficial during the perimenopause, and also a number of complementary therapies which are gaining in popularity. We will look in more detail at these options in *Managing the menopause*.

## TREATMENT OPTIONS FOR THE MENOPAUSE

■ **Lifestyle changes**
  - Eating a healthy, balanced diet
  - Exercising (e.g. weight-bearing exercise like walking or jogging, resistance exercise using weights)
  - Avoiding the things that can bring on your symptoms

■ **Hormone-based treatments**
  - HRT (oestrogen-only, combined sequential or combined continuous; see page 100)
  - Tibolone (Livial®)
  - Phyto-oestrogens (naturally occurring chemicals found in many plant-based foods)
  - Testosterone

■ **Drugs to reduce hot flushes and sweating**
  - Clonidine (Dixarit®, Catapres®)
  - Selective serotonin receptor inhibitors (SSRIs)

■ **Complementary therapies**
  - Herbal remedies
  - Homeopathy
  - Reflexology
  - Hypnosis
  - Acupuncture
  - Aromatherapy
  - Yoga

■ **Treatments for menorrhagia** *(regular but particularly heavy periods, experienced by many women in the run-up to the menopause)*
  - Non-steroidal anti-inflammatory drugs (NSAIDs)
  - Tranexamic acid (Cyklokapron®)
  - Etamsylate (Dicynene®)
  - Progestogen-only therapy (Mirena®)
  - Surgery (e.g. hysterectomy)

All of these therapies are covered in more detail later on in *Managing the menopause.*

■ **Treatments for psychological symptoms**
  – Psychotherapy, counselling
  – Antidepressant drugs[*]

■ **Treatments for urogenital symptoms**
  *(physical symptoms affecting the urinary system and genitalia)*
  – Vaginal lubricants/moisturisers (KY Jelly® or Replens®)
  – Incontinence medications
  – Antibiotics for bladder infections.

[*]If your doctor prescribes you an antidepressant, it does not mean that he thinks your symptoms are 'all in your head'. These can be very effective at stabilising blood vessels and reducing the frequency of hot flushes.

For more information see
**Depression**

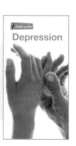

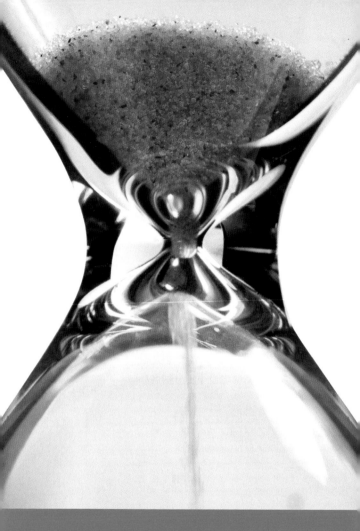

**Why now?**

## WHY NOW?

The menopause happens to all women, but at different ages. What determines when you will have your menopause and does it matter?

You might be surprised to hear that, despite the many improvements in our diet, lifestyle, living conditions and general health, the average age of the menopause has not really changed in centuries.

With the average age of the menopause reported to be 51 years, a woman in the UK can expect to spend over a third of her lifetime postmenopause. However, 100 years ago, the average life expectancy for a woman was only about 50. Not only was the menopause an event that many women never experienced, but even if they did, they would not have expected to live for very long afterwards. As a result, the possible health problems that can occur following sustained low levels of oestrogen that typify postmenopausal life were simply not an issue at this time.

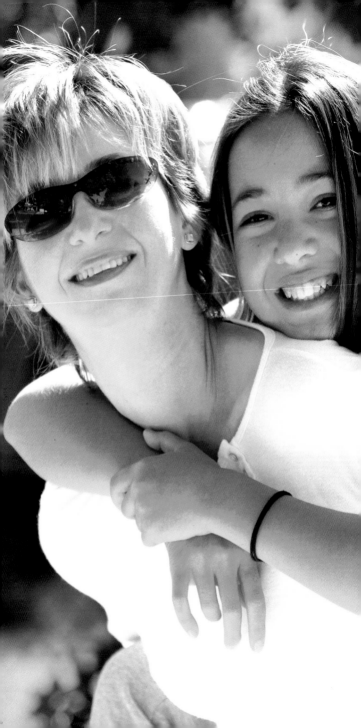

## MENOPAUSE OCCURS WHEN THE OVARIES FAIL

As we saw in *The basics* (page 18), menopause occurs when the ovaries can no longer respond to hormonal signals being sent from the brain (i.e. FSH and LH). These signals are trying to tell the ovaries to produce oestrogen and progesterone and to keep the menstrual cycle running, but the ovaries fail to respond. So why do they begin to fail? There are two main reasons that this might happen.

1.  The ovaries fail as a consequence of getting older (**primary ovarian failure**).

2.  The ovaries fail as a consequence of some other health problem or its treatment (**secondary ovarian failure**).

Possible causes of secondary ovarian failure (that may damage the ovaries and make them more susceptible to failure) include:

■ radiotherapy or chemotherapy for cancer

■ hysterectomy without removal of the ovaries

■ certain infections, such as tuberculosis and mumps.

The age at which your mother had her menopause can often give you some indication of the approximate age at which you might experience yours.

In the case of secondary ovarian failure, it is often quite easy to pinpoint the exact time of menopause and to understand why it has happened. What is less clear is what determines when your ovaries will 'spontaneously' stop producing enough oestrogen and progesterone to keep the menstrual cycle running normally. In most women, primary ovarian failure will occur around the age of 51. It is generally considered that having your menopause at any age between 45 and 55 years is normal. For some women, however, the menopause can come unusually early or late.

## PREMATURE MENOPAUSE

A menopause occurring before the age of 45 is considered early, but **premature menopause** is usually defined as that occurring before the age of 40. Sometimes, premature menopause is also referred to as premature ovarian failure, or POF, because this is the problem that has caused the menopause to come early. It is important to note, however, that POF and premature menopause are not necessarily always the same. Not all cases of POF are permanent – in some cases, ovarian function can be restored and periods can return. As we have seen, the menopause is defined by your very last menstrual period, and this can only occur when POF is permanent.

### SOME STATISTICS ON PREMATURE MENOPAUSE

- Around 1 in every 100 women under 40 have had their menopause
- Around 1 in every 1,000 women under 30 have had their menopause
- Around 1 in every 10,000 women under 20 have had their menopause.

*Source: www.daisynetwork.org.uk*
The Daisy Network Premature Menopause Support Group

You may be more likely to have a premature menopause under the following circumstances.

■ **There are abnormalities in your chromosomes**

Chromosomes are the tiny strands of DNA (deoxyribonucleic acid) in each of your cells that carry your genes. In most of the cells in your body, you have 23 pairs of chromosomes, and one of these pairs holds the sex chromosomes which determine whether you are male or female. Men have an X and a Y chromosome, whereas women have two X chromosomes. However, if there is a defect in one of these X chromosomes (leading to a condition known as 'fragile X syndrome'), you can be born with fewer eggs in your ovaries and as a result are likely to experience an early menopause. Similarly, if part or all of one of the X chromosome is missing (a condition known as Turner's syndrome), you are also likely to experience an early menopause and in some cases you may actually never have menstrual periods at all. In addition, some women are born with three X chromosomes rather than two (a condition known as the triple X syndrome), and this can also encourage a premature menopause.

**You have an autoimmune disease**
Your body's immune system protects you
against 'foreign invaders' such as bacteria, and
therefore prevents infection and disease.
However, if you have an autoimmune disease,
your immune system mistakenly attacks part of
your own body by developing antibodies
against it. Examples of autoimmune diseases
include multiple sclerosis (where your immune
system attacks your nervous system) and
rheumatoid arthritis (where the immune
system attacks the lining of your joints). If you
have an autoimmune condition, or a close
family member does, it is possible that you will
have antibodies against your own ovaries,
uterus lining or even the hormones controlling
your menstrual cycle.

**You have polycystic ovary syndrome**
(a condition in which the ovaries contain
numerous fluid-filled sacs [cysts]). Polycystic
ovaries are common, occurring in one-in-four
to -five women during their reproductive years.

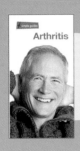

For more information see
**Arthritis**

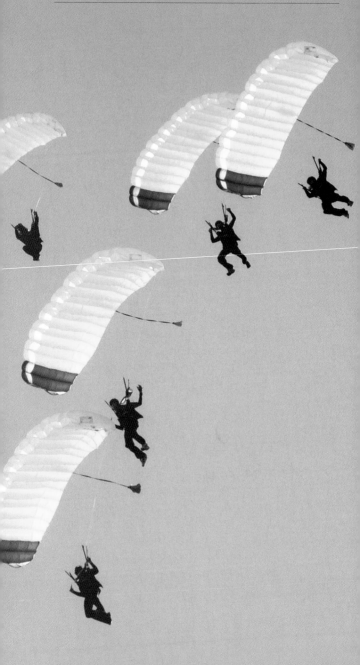

### ■ You have had a hysterectomy

There are numerous reasons for having a hysterectomy and it remains one of the most common types of surgery. It is estimated that, by the age of 55, one-in-five women will have had a hysterectomy. The most common reasons include:

– heavy or irregular menstrual bleeding
– large, painful or damaged fibroids (non cancerous growths)
– cancer of the uterus, ovaries, or cervix
– uterine prolapse (a condition in which the uterus starts to move down into the vagina)
– endometriosis (a condition in which tissue resembling the lining of the uterus grows in the abdomen, such as the pelvis, ovaries, bladder and bowels. These growths react to oestrogen and progesterone in the same way as the endometrium [the lining of the uterus], and so bleed internally during a menstrual period.)

If your ovaries are removed during the procedure (oophorectomy), then your menopause will be immediate and inevitable. Following an oophorectomy, you might expect to start experiencing menopausal symptoms within a few days. If you have a hysterectomy in which the ovaries were left intact, your ovaries may continue to function normally and then fail close to the normal age of 51. However, there is an increased chance of premature ovarian failure (POF) in the years following a hysterectomy.

**TYPES OF HYSTERECTOMY**

■ Partial/subtotal hysterectomy
The body of the uterus is removed but the cervix is left intact, attached to the vagina.

■ Total hysterectomy
The uterus and cervix are removed (this is the most common form of hysterectomy).

■ Total hysterectomy with unilateral salpingo-oophorectomy
The uterus, cervix and one fallopian tube and ovary are removed.

■ Total hysterectomy with bilateral salpingo-oophorectomy
The uterus, cervix and both fallopian tubes and ovaries are removed.

■ Wertheim's/radical hysterectomy
The uterus, cervix, upper part of the vagina, fallopian tubes and supporting tissues are removed, often with some lymph nodes (the bean-shaped structures of the immune system that help the body to fight infections) removed too.

### ■ You are being treated with radiotherapy or chemotherapy

These treatments are designed to kill cancer cells, but unfortunately are also likely to damage your ovaries. This is one cause of premature ovarian failure. In some cases, menstrual periods may just stop temporarily and return when treatment is stopped, but other times the change is permanent, and therefore marks the menopause. Even if periods do return, a woman is often infertile following radiotherapy or chemotherapy. As a precaution, many women opt to have some eggs frozen before undergoing treatment.

### ■ You have a family history of premature menopause

In general, it seems that many women have their menopause at a similar age to their mother, so there is probably something in your genes that helps determine your menopausal age. Therefore, if your mother, or indeed a grandmother or sister, for example, has had a premature menopause, you may be at increased risk of having one yourself. However, to put this in perspective, studies have reported that only about one-in-twenty women who have a premature menopause actually have a family history of it.

■ **You are a smoker**
There is evidence that smoking increases your
risk of premature menopause. The longer you
have been smoking, and the heavier a smoker
you are, the more impact this may have on
your time of menopause.

■ **You, or your mother, have had viral
infections**
Certain viral infections, such as mumps, may
affect ovarian function and put you at risk of
premature menopause. Also, if your mother
suffered one of these infections whilst
pregnant with you, it is possible that this
could have affected the development of your
ovaries and put you at increased risk of
premature menopause.

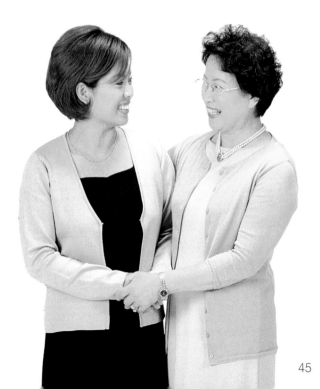

## LATE MENOPAUSE

By the age of 54, four out of five women will have
had their menopause. However, if the menopause
is delayed until after the age of 55, it is generally
considered to be late. You might be more likely to
have a late menopause if you are overweight. As
we have seen, most of your oestrogen is made in
your ovaries. However, a small amount is also
made in other parts of the body, including fat
cells. If you are obese (i.e. your body mass index
or BMI is over 30), you will be exposed to higher
levels of oestrogen throughout your life.
Therefore, as well as increasing your risk of
serious health problems, such as breast cancer
and heart disease, being overweight can also
delay your menopause.

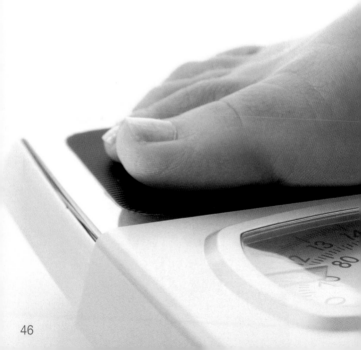

## CALCULATE YOUR OWN BODY MASS INDEX (BMI)

It's very simple to work out your own BMI, to see whether your weight has delayed your menopause. Grab a tape measure, a set of bathroom scales and a calculator and follow these two steps.

■ Measure your height in metres. Multiply this number by itself and write down the answer, for example:

**1.80 (metres) × 1.80 = 3.24**

■ Measure your weight in kilograms. Divide it by the number you wrote down in the first step, for example:

**80 (kilograms) ÷ 3.24 = 24.7**

*The number you get is your BMI.* As a general rule, for adults aged over 20, the BMI relates to the following:

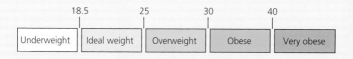

| | 18.5 | 25 | 30 | 40 |
|---|---|---|---|---|
| Underweight | Ideal weight | Overweight | Obese | Very obese |

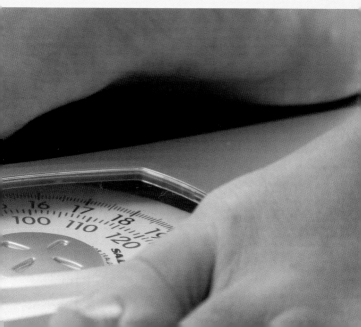

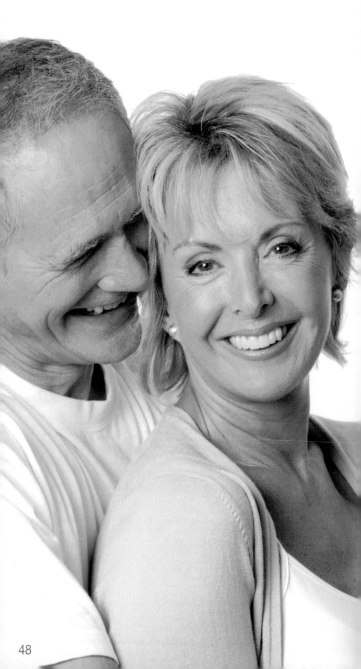

## HOW WILL THE MENOPAUSE AFFECT ME?

The menopause is not nicknamed 'the change of life' for nothing. Whatever age you experience it, it has important implications that may affect your day-to-day life. Some women sail through the menopause without being troubled by symptoms or being bothered by the arrival of the end of their reproductive life. Indeed many women welcome the fact that they are no longer at risk of becoming pregnant and can therefore enjoy love-making without worrying about contraception.

For others, particularly if it is early and unexpected, the menopause can be a traumatic and uncomfortable experience. Being aware of how the menopause might affect you, can help you to deal with the changes that you may experience. If you recognise why you are feeling the way you are, it should be easier to ask your doctor for help and advice.

We have already looked at the symptoms that you might expect to experience around the time of your menopause. Some, such as the hot flushes and irritability, will most likely have resolved by a year or two after your last menstrual period. Others, such as sexual problems and incontinence, may last much longer. These symptoms can really affect your quality of life, in a way that people who have not been through the menopause might not appreciate. If you do experience problems with excessive sweating, for example, you may find that it limits your ability to take regular exercise. Hot flushes may cause embarrassment in public. There is also a considerable emotional burden involved in reaching the menopause too.

It is easy for someone else to say "well, it happens to every woman eventually, doesn't it?", but this probably won't help you if you are feeling distressed about reaching the end of your reproductive life or having reached a significant landmark in the ageing process. Other factors may be coming into play at this time too, such as the upheaval of your children leaving home or perhaps losing a parent. It can be a very difficult time.

These negative feelings can be amplified further if you are struck by an unexpectedly premature menopause. In this case, certain issues become more of a problem, such as premature infertility and an increased risk of complications such as osteoporosis. It is vitally important that you try and stay positive about all of these hurdles. Your doctor will be able to advise you on all of the options available to you to make your situation as comfortable as possible.

Believe it or not, there can be some positive aspects to the menopause. It can be a trigger to push you into adopting an improved, healthier lifestyle, with a better diet and more regular exercise. All of these will be important in warding off the possible health problems that can come into play after your menopause. Many women experience heavy, and perhaps unpredictable menstrual periods in the run up to their menopause, and feel tremendous relief when they stop. Even if the periods have remained fairly regular and of normal volume, there can still be a sense of liberation when they eventually stop.

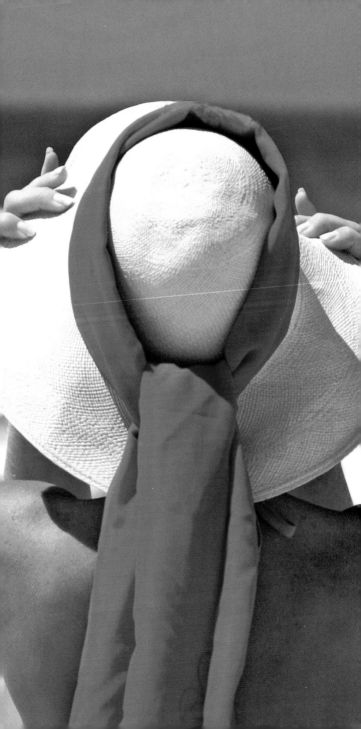

## HOW WILL THE MENOPAUSE AFFECT MY FAMILY?

Many people, including other women, have very little understanding about what happens around the time of the menopause and how it will affect you. The fact that you are reading this book should help you to begin to understand what to expect. It should also reassure you that if you are experiencing symptoms and negative feelings, these will usually improve with time. However, in the meantime, there are plenty of good reasons that you may wish to seek medical help, and you should certainly not be ashamed in doing so.

If you are finding the time around your menopause difficult, it will probably really help both you and your family if they have some idea of what you are going through. It may be difficult for them to understand why your behaviour is changing or why you appear to be unwell more often. Your children, in particular, might find it quite upsetting. Even if they are grown up and have moved away, you are still their mum! Try to explain how you are feeling to your family, and offer reasons if you feel too uncomfortable to join in with certain activities. This will help them to understand that you are not just being 'difficult', and they may be able to reassure you. Encouraging them to read this book may help!

Your partner will need to be understanding and patient if you are suffering from discomfort during sexual intercourse or if you have a reduced libido or interest in love-making. Also, if you are having difficulty sleeping, due to night sweats, for example, this will probably affect your partner's sleeping patterns too. You should reassure them that these problems should resolve with time, and encourage them to help you explore treatment options with your doctor.

Finally, as difficult as it may seem, try and focus on the positive aspects of the menopause. It will be important for you to have a healthy diet and to take regular exercise throughout your postmenopausal years. It is much easier to stick to these strategies when there is someone else doing them with you, so try to encourage your partner, children and friends to join in.

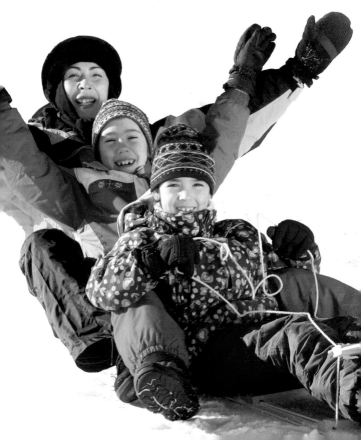

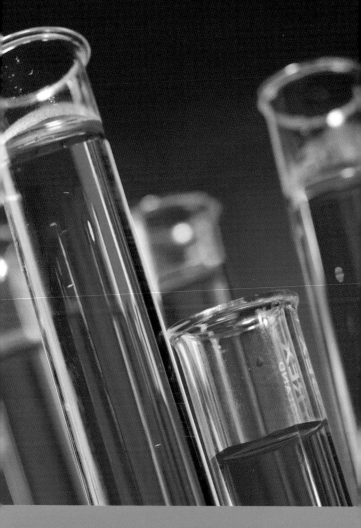

# Simple
# science

# SIMPLE SCIENCE

Most of the changes that you go through around the time of your menopause are due to falling levels of the hormone oestrogen.

In *What happens before the menopause?* (page 6), we saw how the fluctuating levels of the four hormones follicle-stimulating hormone (FSH), luteinising hormone (LH), oestrogen and progesterone regulate the menstrual cycle and cause you to have menstrual periods. We have also established that your body stops undergoing menstrual cycles at the menopause because your ovaries are no longer producing sufficient oestrogen and progesterone to keep the cycle turning over.

So, we now understand the science behind the most obvious change that happens at menopause – the stopping of periods.

But women going through the menopause are often bombarded with recommendations for drugs, lifestyle changes and alternative treatments, and none of these were designed with the intention of bringing the periods back – not many women would claim to miss them! They can't bring back your ability to reproduce, either. It is the symptoms that can come with the menopause, and the possible health problems arising from it, that are deserving of treatment. In order to understand how these treatments are working, we need to look at how the changes that occur at the menopause can cause such physical and emotional upheaval.

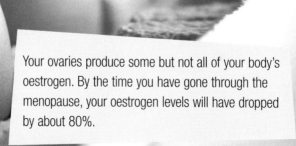

Your ovaries produce some but not all of your body's oestrogen. By the time you have gone through the menopause, your oestrogen levels will have dropped by about 80%.

## THE MENOPAUSE AND VASOMOTOR SYMPTOMS

In biological terms, the word vasomotor means 'affecting the calibre of a blood vessel' – in other words, altering the diameter of the tubes through which the blood flows. Under normal circumstances, your body uses your blood vessels as a means of temperature control. When blood flows around your extremities (e.g. in your arms, legs, fingers, toes), it cools because it is reasonably close to your skin. When this cooled blood then returns to your 'core' (deeper inside your body), it reduces your core body temperature. Because of this, if your body temperature is getting too low, the blood vessels in your extremities get narrower (constrict), which reduces the amount of blood that can flow around these areas. In contrast, when your core temperature is increasing, the blood vessels in your extremities get wider (dilate), allowing more blood to flow around these areas and cool down.

It is thought that falling levels of oestrogen are responsible for problems with the dilation and constriction of blood vessels, and so cause malfunction of the body's temperature regulation system. This would certainly explain the hot flushes and abnormal levels of sweating associated with the menopause. Palpitations, dizziness and headaches may also be related to problems with the way in which the blood vessels dilate or constrict.

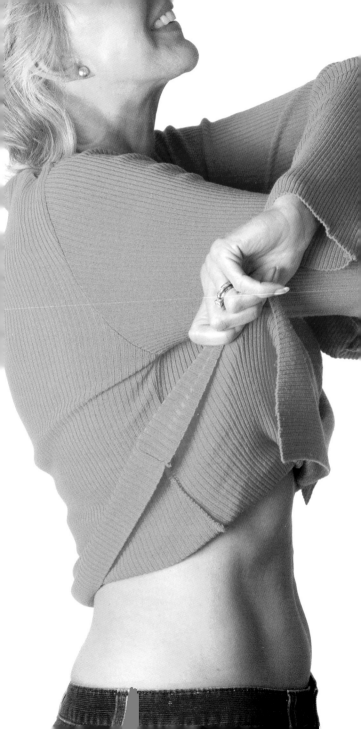

Scientists are also discovering that there is substantial interplay between oestrogen and a chemical called serotonin. Problems with the serotonin system are known to be a factor in causing depression, and because of the emerging links with oestrogen, it is possible that they may also play a role in causing menopausal symptoms too. Drugs that are used as antidepressants because they affect the amount of serotonin available in the brain (selective serotonin reuptake inhibitors [SSRIs]) also appear to be effective in controlling hot flushes.

It may seem strange to treat menopausal symptoms with the same drugs that are used to treat depression, but rest assured if your doctor prescribes you an antidepressant, it does not mean that he thinks your symptoms are 'all in your head'.

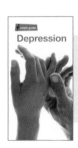

For more information see
**Depression**

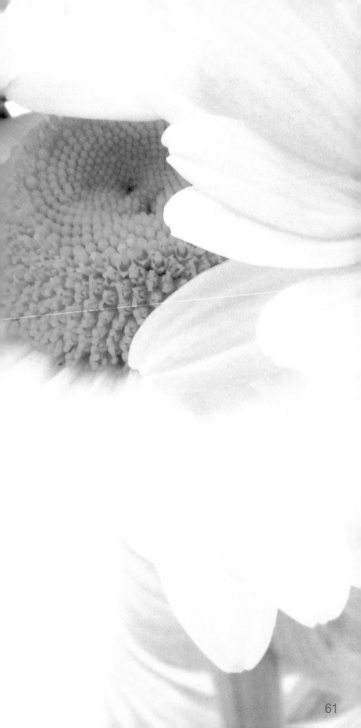

**The menopause and urogenital symptoms**

Urogenital symptoms are those symptoms that affect the urinary system and the genitalia. Oestrogen exerts control over these areas of your body, and when levels of this hormone start to get low in the lead up to the menopause, this is likely to lead to a few noticeable changes.

■ Oestrogen is required for the skin and supporting tissues in the vulva (the external female genitalia – clitoris, vaginal lips and opening to the vagina) and the vagina to remain strong and elastic. When there is little oestrogen available, these areas of skin become thin and the vulva can lose some of its plumpness.

■ Oestrogen also promotes the production of mucus in the vagina by mucus glands. Reduced mucus production after the menopause causes vaginal dryness. This, together with the fragility of the skin around the vulva and vagina, can result in soreness during and after sexual intercourse.

■ Oestrogen has considerable control over the condition of your urogenital system. In particular, it stops the pH from getting too high. In other words, oestrogen ensures that the inside of your vagina, bladder and urethra is slightly acidic. This acidic environment is not a good environment for bacteria to grow, and so oestrogen helps to protect against infection of the vagina and urinary tract. After the menopause, you might be at increased risk of such infections.

■ Due to the changing environment in the vagina caused by falling oestrogen levels, vaginal discharge may also occur. Losing small amounts of fluid from your vagina, usually clear or milky and odourless, is normal. However, after the menopause you might find that your vaginal discharge becomes more watery, discoloured, and may be a little smelly.

■ The muscles and ligaments which support the uterus and bladder are sensitive to oestrogen. When oestrogen levels fall, these muscles and ligaments weaken, and the uterus may begin to prolapse (move down into the vagina). You may also feel that the walls of your vagina are becoming more floppy.

■ Urinary incontinence is a common problem amongst postmenopausal women. Falling levels of oestrogen can weaken the pelvic floor muscles, which support the bladder and the urethra, and make it difficult for you to stop urine leaking from your bladder. There are many other factors, however, that can contribute to urinary incontinence, such as pregnancy, side-effects of drugs taken for other conditions, constipation, surgery and general weakening of muscles with age.

■ Given the right treatment, urinary incontinence can be controlled effectively and need not impinge on your quality of life. We will cover the management options later on in the *Managing the menopause* section.

## THE PSYCHOLOGICAL EFFECTS OF THE MENOPAUSE

It is quite possible that you will experience psychological symptoms to some extent in the time surrounding the menopause. Most commonly, these might include irritability, mood swings, depression and forgetfulness. To a large extent, these feelings may simply be due to the emotional burden of the physical symptoms that you might be experiencing. There is not really any conclusive evidence that the changing levels of hormones around the time of the menopause can have any noticeable effect on your mood or behaviour. However, by creating physical symptoms at a time which can already be emotionally draining, falling oestrogen levels are probably responsible for indirectly affecting mood.

The impact that urogenital symptoms can have on sexual function can be particularly distressing, causing feelings of embarrassment and inadequacy in some women. However, testosterone is also important in this respect. Although usually considered to be a male hormone, testosterone is produced by your ovaries prior to menopause and is important for maintaining your sex drive. When the ovaries fail at menopause, testosterone production drops in the same way as oestrogen, and this can result in reduced libido. When given as a drug treatment, small amounts of testosterone can help to restore this.

## MENOPAUSE AND BONE STRENGTH

Osteoporosis is a potentially serious disease in which bones become less dense and therefore weaker and prone to fractures. The most important risk factor for osteoporosis in women is the menopause, and this is directly related to the drop in oestrogen levels that occurs at this time. You may not be aware of this, but bone is actually living tissue, and is constantly being 'turned over'. Old bone is broken down (in a process known as resorption) and new bone is created in its place.

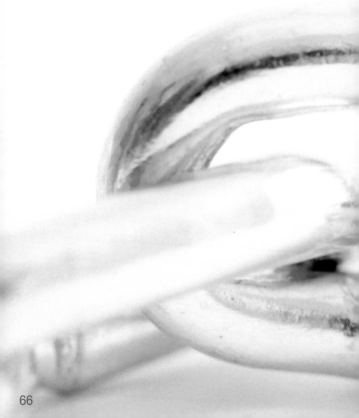

Oestrogen has a crucial role in limiting the amount of bone resorption. When the levels of oestrogen start to fall in the period leading up to the menopause, the rate of bone resorption starts to exceed the rate at which new bone is formed in its place. As a result, there is a net loss of bone, and if the density of the bones falls to a particularly low level, this is known as osteoporosis. Other factors, such as a family history of osteoporosis, a history of poor diet or eating disorders, smoking or drug treatment, can affect your risk of developing this condition, However, the menopause increases every woman's risk of osteoporosis.

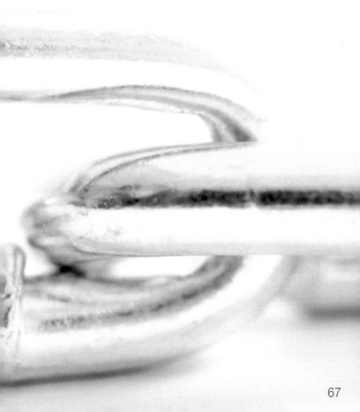

## MENOPAUSE, BODY WEIGHT AND THE CARDIOVASCULAR SYSTEM

Premenopausal women have a considerably smaller risk of cardiovascular disease (such as heart attacks and stroke) than men of the same age. However, following the menopause, a woman's risk of these problems starts to increase significantly. There are a number of potential reasons for this, including problems with dilation and constriction of blood vessels that we looked at earlier. Low levels of oestrogen can also cause the blood to become more 'sticky', increasing the risk of clots. Furthermore, the menopause affects cholesterol levels, causing an increase in the level of 'bad' (LDL, low density lipoprotein) cholesterol, and thus increasing the risk of heart disease.

Another important factor in increasing the risk of cardiovascular disease is the effect of menopause on body weight. Many women find that they put on weight after the menopause,

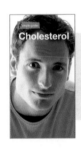

For more information see
**Cholesterol**

particularly around the abdominal area. It is this kind of fat distribution which puts you at risk of heart and circulation problems. Other factors which lead to increased weight around the time of the menopause, such as taking less exercise, losing muscle and having a slower metabolism, will also contribute to the increased cardiovascular risk.

## MENOPAUSE AND BREAST CANCER

This may be a hard one to get your head around. Although most cases of breast cancer occur in postmenopausal women, having a later menopause increases your risk of breast cancer. Confused? Have a look at the graph. The risk of breast cancer increases with age, doubling approximately every 10 years, but once you hit menopause, this age-related increase in risk starts to slow down. It is generally accepted that your risk of getting breast cancer is related to the extent to which your breast tissue is exposed to oestrogen throughout your life. Women who have a particularly late menopause (for example over the age of 55) or a particularly early menarche (before the age of 12) are at slightly higher risk of breast cancer than those who have their menopause earlier. These women have had a greater than average lifetime exposure to oestrogen.

Other factors such as being older than 35 when you have your first child, or indeed never having children, can also increase your risk of breast cancer, as can having a family history of the disease and being overweight after the menopause. In keeping with the evidence that greater oestrogen exposure increases your risk of breast cancer, there is evidence that receiving HRT for a number of years can also increases your risk – we will look at this particular issue in *Managing the menopause* page 112.

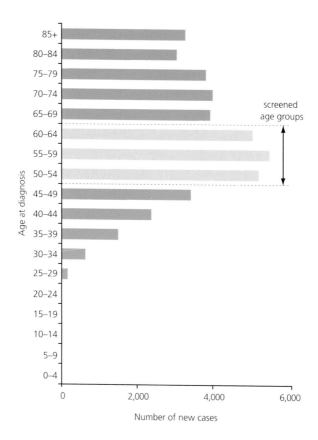

NUMBER OF NEW CASES OF BREAST CANCER
IN THE UK, BY AGE, IN 2002.
*Source: Cancer Research UK, http://info.cancerresearchuk.org*

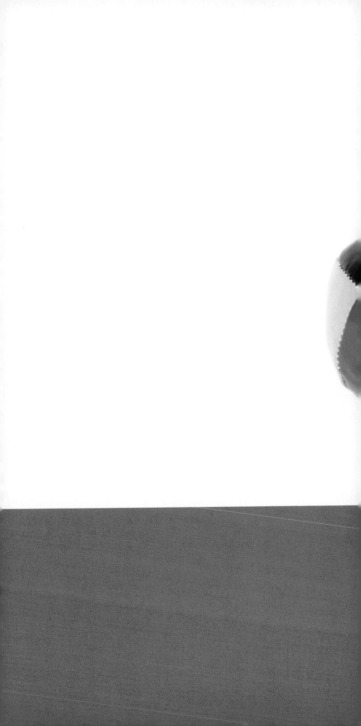

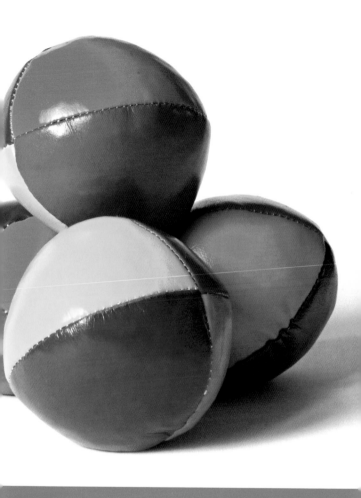

# Managing the
# menopause

# MANAGING THE MENOPAUSE

The menopause experience varies a great deal from woman to woman. The amount of support that you receive is very much up to you, but it is important for you to be aware of all the options available.

### HOW DO I KNOW WHEN I HAVE REACHED THE MENOPAUSE?

As we have seen, the menopause itself is your last menstrual period. There are a number of signs that can suggest that the menopause is on its way.

- Your periods are becoming irregular.

- Your periods are becoming abnormally light or heavy.

- You are beginning to experience symptoms. We have already looked at the range of symptoms that the menopause can bring on (see *The basics* page 20). Roughly two-thirds of women will experience symptoms around the time of their menopause. Although the symptoms are mostly brought on by hormonal changes, they can also be affected by diet, level of exercise and medications.

If you are approaching the typical age at which you might expect to reach the menopause (about 51), these signs will not be unexpected. If you are much younger, however, you are probably less likely to realise what these signs may be telling you.

**WHAT IS A HEAVY PERIOD?**

Every woman knows how heavy their own periods normally are, but some variation between periods is to be expected. How do you know when your periods are 'abnormally heavy'?

- You need to double up on sanitary protection (towels and tampons, for example) or need to change your sanitary towels at least every 2 hours.

- You notice clots in the blood you lose during your periods.

- Your periods restrict your daily life. For example, they prevent you from going out, or present difficulties at work.

- You start to suffer from anaemia. You may feel dizzy and tired, and look pale, due to a shortage of red blood cells.

It is possible to test for the menopause, by measuring the level of follicle-stimulating hormone (FSH) in your blood or urine. As we have seen, when your ovaries start to fail, they stop responding to the FSH and luteinising hormone (LH) signals sent from the brain. The brain generates more FSH and LH in an attempt to get the message across, and the increased level of FSH can therefore be used as a marker for the menopause. It is important to remember, particularly if you buy a home-testing kit rather than having the test done by a doctor, that FSH levels fluctuate a great deal throughout the month anyway. They can also be affected by medications such as the oral contraceptive pill and some antidepressants. In normal circumstances, your doctor would not rely on the results of such a test

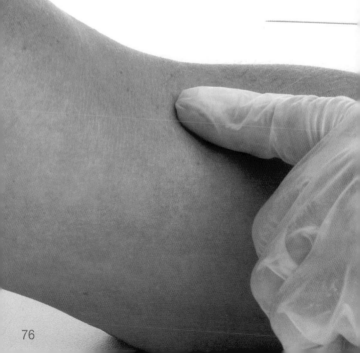

to determine whether you were close to the menopause – your symptom history and pattern of recent periods are far more important factors. A doctor would probably only use the test if you have had a hysterectomy but your ovaries were left in place, as a means of identifying whether the ovaries have failed (as you won't have periods after a hysterectomy so can't use menstrual periods as a sign of whether your ovaries are working!).

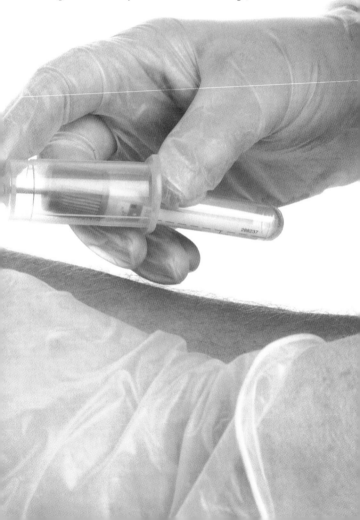

## WHAT ELSE COULD IT BE?

There are a number of other health problems that may cause symptoms that resemble those associated with the menopause. On the one hand, you may worry unduly that you are suffering from one of these conditions, not realising that you are actually reaching the menopause, particularly if it has arrived early. On the other hand, it is important not to assume that any symptoms around your late 40s or early 50s can be simply put down to the menopause. If for any reason your symptoms are not what you expected, it is important to consult your doctor, who will be able to exclude any more serious underlying conditions. Other conditions that may cause symptoms similar to the menopause include:

- pregnancy

- thyroid disease

- ovarian cancer

- polycystic ovarian syndrome (a condition in which the ovaries contain numerous fluid-filled sacs [cysts])

- hyperprolactinaemia (an abnormally high level of a hormone called prolactin in the blood)

- pituitary disorders (problems with the pituitary gland in the brain that produces, amongst other hormones, FSH and LH)

- Cushing's disease (caused by a tumour in the pituitary gland, which results in excessive production of a hormone called cortisol).

## THE FEMALE ATHLETE TRIAD

The female athlete triad refers to three related health issues:

- eating disorders
- absence of periods (amenorrhoea)
- osteoporosis.

This triad of problems is particularly common amongst female athletes, as the name suggests, but can also affect any woman who is excessively concerned with their weight and body shape. These three problems can occur when a woman uses potentially harmful, and often ineffective, methods to achieve their 'ideal' shape and weight. Excessive exercise and eating disorders can reduce a woman's oestrogen levels, causing problems with her menstrual cycle, as demonstrated by amenorrhoea, and increasing the risk of osteoporosis in later life.

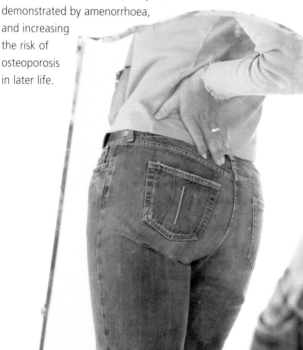

The defining feature of the menopause is, of course, the stopping of menstrual periods. A number of factors, other than spontaneous primary ovarian failure at the menopause, can cause periods to stop temporarily. These include:

■ excessive and rapid weight change

■ excessive exercise

■ recent discontinuation of the oral contraceptive pill.

Conversely, a common experience for many women in the run up to the menopause is that periods become heavier than normal. There are a number of possible reasons for heavy periods (menorrhagia), other than the menopause. These include:

■ fibroids (benign lumps in the muscle wall of the uterus)

■ endometriosis (patches of endometrial tissue growing outside the uterus, for example in the ovaries)

■ infection of the uterus, vagina or cervix

■ polyps (benign growths on the cervix or uterus).

A 'normal' period for most women lasts 3–7 days, and involves the loss of about 4–12 teaspoonfuls of blood (that's between 20 and 60 mL).

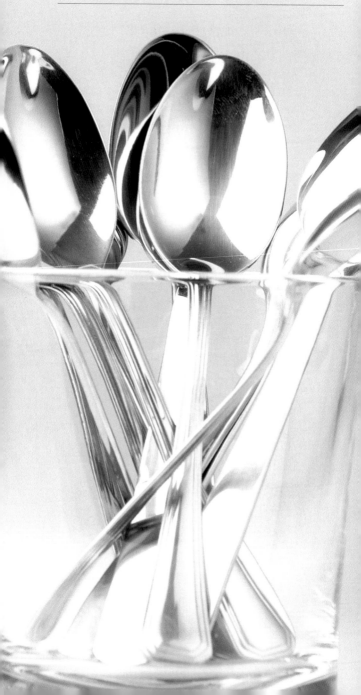

## WHEN SHOULD I SEE A DOCTOR?

This book has highlighted a lot of symptoms and potential complications of the menopause, because it is important that you are aware of them, understand them, and know how you can best manage them. However, it is important to remember that plenty of women find the so-called 'change of life' a very easy transition which only has a minimal impact on their lives. There is no need for every woman who goes through the menopause to consult her doctor.

### Excluding other health problems

You may wish to see your doctor if you think you have reached your menopause, just to reassure yourself that your 'diagnosis' is correct and there are no other underlying health problems. Your doctor will be quite happy to see you and to answer any questions you might have.

There are certain situations in which you definitely should consult a doctor when your periods appear to have stopped, so that they can exclude other possible reasons for the amenorrhoea.

- Your periods have stopped but there is a possibility that you are pregnant.
- Your periods stopped for a few months and then started again.
- Your periods seem to have stopped and you are under the age of 45.
- Your periods have stopped and you are experiencing unusual symptoms, such as a bloated or swollen abdomen.
- You have irregular bleeding or spotting or you bleed after intercourse.

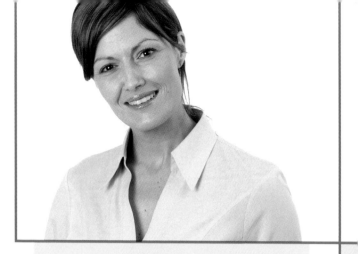

### GP

As your GP, I will probably be your first port of call if you have any concerns or uncertainties about reaching the menopause. I can help you to determine whether the symptoms and/or changes you are experiencing are indeed due to the menopause. I can prescribe you medications if we decide between us that this is the best option, but I can also offer advice, reassurance and explanation of anything you are unsure about.

If your menopause is to be brought on immediately by surgery, this will be carried out in a hospital. However, I can support you in the lead up to your operation and will provide ongoing care afterwards to help you and your family to adjust.

The menopause is a very individual experience, and we can work together to make sure that we make it as easy as possible for you, as well as making sure that we give you the best chance for a healthy postmenopausal life.

83

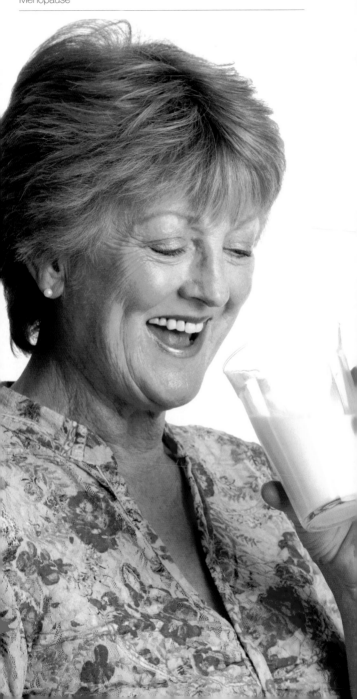

**Preventing postmenopausal complications**

You may also wish to consult a doctor if you simply want some advice on how to stay healthy after your menopause. This may involve basic dietary advice and exercise regimens, but is more critical if you are considered to be at particular risk of the potential complications of menopause, such as osteoporosis and cardiovascular disease.

## OSTEOPOROSIS

As we saw in *Simple science* (page 66), the drop in oestrogen levels around the time of menopause makes your bones deteriorate more quickly, and so your risk of osteoporosis will steadily increase from this point.

You might be at increased risk of osteoporosis if:

- there is a history of bone fractures, particularly hip fracture, after the age of 50 in your family

- you have a petite frame (a BMI below 19)

- you smoke

- you get very little exercise

- you have been using oral steroid drugs for other conditions (e.g. asthma)

- you have had an eating disorder in the past or your periods have stopped previously when you were not pregnant

- you have one of a number of other conditions (e.g. rheumatoid arthritis or liver/kidney disease) which increase your risk of osteoporosis.

## CARDIOVASCULAR DISEASE

You are considered to be at an increased risk of cardiovascular disease if:

- you are overweight, particularly if your fat is primarily located around your waist; this 'apple' body shape puts you most at risk of cardiovascular disease
- there is a history of cardiovascular disease in your family
- you smoke or drink too much alcohol (more than 1 or 2 units a day)
- you have high blood cholesterol
- you have high blood pressure
- you get very little exercise
- you have diabetes.

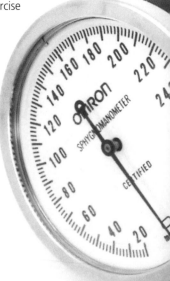

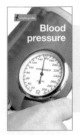

For more information see
**Blood pressure**

As we saw in *Simple science* (page 58), some of the changes that occur around the menopause, such as blood vessels becoming less efficient at altering their calibre and the body developing a tendency to store fat around the abdomen, can put you at increased risk of cardiovascular disease. If some of the risk factors listed above apply to you, it is important to consult your doctor as you may need drug treatments or to make lifestyle changes in order to protect your heart.

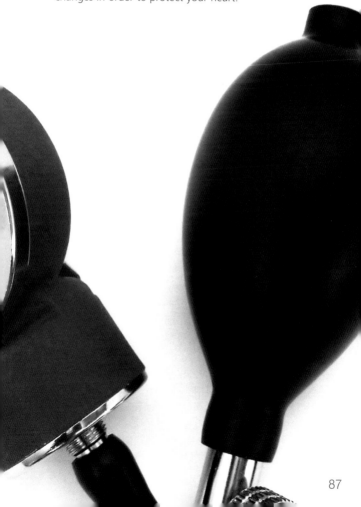

### Relief of symptoms

The most likely reason for you to go and see your doctor when going through the menopause are the symptoms associated with it. If you are experiencing symptoms which are particularly uncomfortable, embarrassing, making your daily life difficult or simply proving too much to deal with, you should consult your doctor. Whilst there are some safety concerns surrounding the long-term use of HRT (over 5 years), use of this treatment for a few years whilst menopausal symptoms are proving a problem can be very effective.

Do not suffer in silence – your perimenopausal years can be made much easier if you are prepared to seek help. There is no shame in going to your doctor about your symptoms – some women get off more lightly at the menopause, whilst others are burdened with troublesome symptoms. If you are in the latter category, there is no need to just grin and bear it!

### THE WELL WOMAN CHECK

Many surgeries, and a lot of private health clinics, offer a check-up known as a Well Woman Check. This is designed to assess your general health and to pick up any potential health problems at an early stage, before you have noticed anything wrong. If you are invited for a Well Woman Check around the time of your menopause, this will provide you with information about your risk of cardiovascular disease, and perhaps osteoporosis, and also help your doctor to establish what action you need to take to ensure that you stay healthy after your menopause.

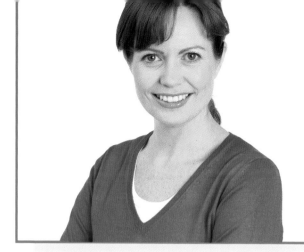

## PRACTICE NURSE

As a practice nurse with a specialist interest in women's health, I work together with the GPs in the practice to provide care and education about the menopause and postmenopausal life. Understanding what is happening and why as you go through this major change is very important, both for you and your family. It will help you to know what to expect as you approach the menopause, as well as teaching you to recognise signs in your postmenopausal life that something might be wrong and you ought to see your GP.

I will be able to talk over with you any medications you are taking, and discuss any worries you have, relating to the use of HRT, for example. I will also be responsible for running Well Woman Checks, which can help you to appreciate your overall level of health and to establish whether you need to make any changes to your lifestyle.

## YOUR LIFESTYLE AFTER THE MENOPAUSE

Ensuring that you have a healthy lifestyle will help your body to adapt to the changes that the menopause brings with it. Not only can your diet and your level of exercise help to control any menopausal symptoms that you might be experiencing, but they can also minimise your risk of future health problems that are associated with postmenopausal hormone levels.

## ADOPT A HEALTHY DIET

It is vital that you maintain a balanced diet that provides you with your daily requirements of calories, but also try not to exceed these allowances.

Note that fats are an important part of your diet, and you would certainly be mistaken to assume that all fats are 'bad'. Try to make sure that you get most of your fat allowance from mono- or polyunsaturated fats, good sources of which include oily fish (e.g. sardines), nuts and seeds, avocados and olive, vegetable and rapeseed oils. These fats are much better for you than the saturated fats that are found in fatty meats, cheese and cream, for example.

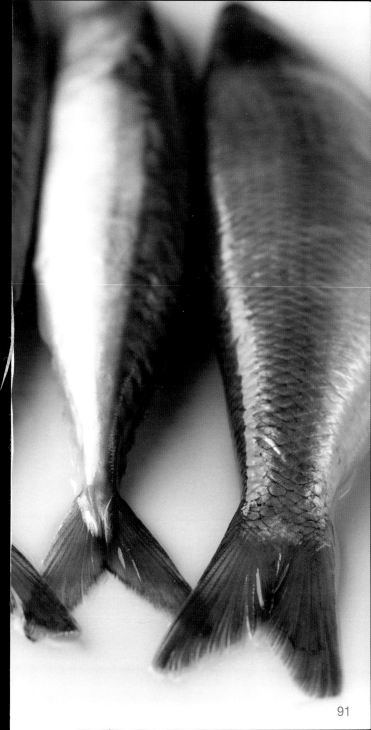

In addition to maintaining a healthy balance of proteins, fats and carbohydrates, a number of nutrients are particularly important as you reach the menopause.

■ **Calcium**

This is vital for bone strength, and with the increased risk of osteoporosis that comes with reaching the menopause, it is important that you give your bones every possible chance to stay strong and healthy. Good sources of calcium include dairy products (e.g. milk, cheese). If you think that this amount of calcium is more than you can reasonably get in your diet, ask your doctor about taking calcium supplements.

■ **Vitamin D**

Like calcium, this is needed for healthy bones and teeth. This is because it helps the body to absorb calcium from food. Most of our vitamin D is made in our skin when it is exposed to sunlight, but a small amount should come from the foods that we eat. As you get older, you may start to expose less skin to sunlight, and you need to make up for this by ensuring that there is sufficient vitamin D in your diet. Good sources of vitamin D include oily fish, such as sardines or mackerel, liver and eggs. Vitamin D supplements are also available and are particularly useful if you do not eat fish.

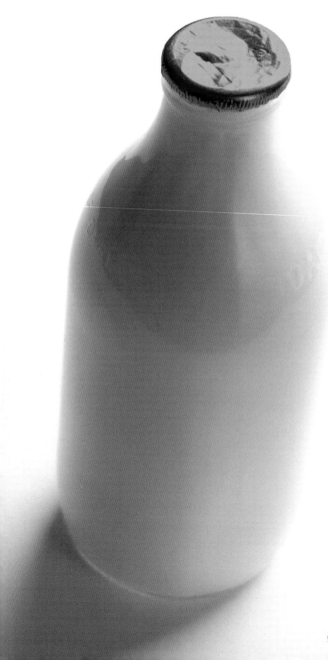

■ **Vitamin E**

When working with other antioxidants in the diet, this may offer some protection against heart problems and may also provide some relief from hot flushes and night sweats. As such, vitamin E can be important for women around the time of their menopause, and it can be found in foods such as nuts, seeds, vegetable oils and cereals, though supplements are available. If you are considering taking vitamin E supplements, however, ask your doctor for advice, as too much vitamin E can be dangerous, particularly if you are taking blood-thinning medications like warfarin.

■ **Phyto-oestrogens**

These are chemicals found in some plants, which, once broken down by the human body after being eaten, act like a weak form of oestrogen. There is some evidence that eating foods rich in phyto-oestrogens, or taking supplements (in the form of red clover pills, for example) may help to reduce hot flushes, headaches, nervousness and sleep problems. Good sources of these chemicals include soya products (e.g. tofu, soya milk), beans, lentils, wheat and celery.

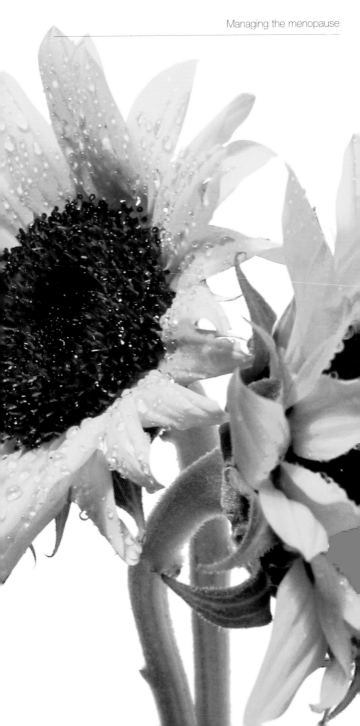

## EXERCISE REGULARLY

Although you may feel restricted by menopause-related problems such as sweating and hot flushes, it is important that you try to maintain a regular programme of weight-bearing exercise. This means that you should support your own body weight whilst carrying out the exercise – running is more effective than cycling or swimming, though any exercise is better than none! The need for exercise to be vigorous and weight-bearing relates to its role in preventing osteoporosis.

Bones that are required to bear weight and experience some impact, as is the case when you are running, are much more likely to stay strong. Resistance exercise (working out with weights) can also help to maintain and can even increase bone mass. Another important reason to partake in regular exercise is to keep your heart healthy and to minimise your risk of developing cardiovascular disease.

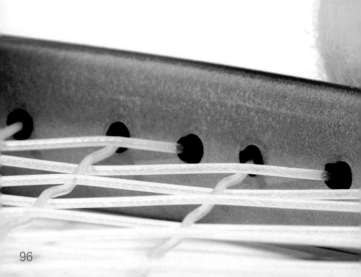

If you find that you have problems with excessive sweating that restricts your level of exercise, it is important to consult your doctor. Developing a lifestyle which involves plenty of exercise is very important at your stage of life, and if troublesome symptoms are preventing this, they need to be dealt with.

## STOP SMOKING

Not only is smoking associated with an earlier menopause it also has serious health implications when you get there. Smoking is bad for your health at the best of times, but smoking and the menopause are a terrible combination. As we have seen, you are at higher risk of osteoporosis and cardiovascular disease once you have passed the menopause, and both of these risks are increased even further if you smoke. If you smoke, try and quit now! Your local NHS Stop Smoking Service can help by putting you in touch with specially trained advisors (call 0800 169 0169). Many practices will be willing to supply nicotine replacement therapy on prescription if you are attending a smoking cessation clinic and trying hard to quit.

## A NOTE ON CONTRACEPTION

One fundamental aspect of the menopause is that it marks the end of your reproductive life.
But a note of caution: as we have seen, it is very difficult to pinpoint exactly when the menopause happens. Remember that menstrual periods can become quite infrequent before stopping altogether and eggs are still released from the ovaries late in the menopausal transition. An unexpected pregnancy late in your reproductive life could be wrought with biological, psychological and social problems so it is very important that you continue to use contraception until you have been at least a year without a period or 2 years if you are under 50. If you are at all unsure, ask your doctor for advice.

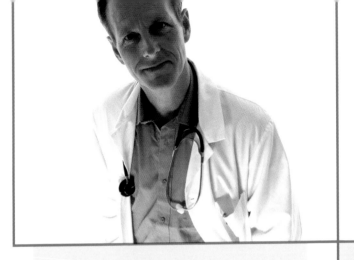

### GYNAECOLOGIST

As a doctor specialising in the female reproductive system, my role is to care for women who have problems that the GP cannot reasonably deal with in the surgery. If you are suffering particularly heavy bleeding, for example, your GP might refer you to me, and if necessary, I can offer you surgical treatments (such as a hysterectomy or endometrial ablation).

I might also become involved in your care if you have an early menopause and wish to pursue IVF treatment in order to have a baby. A number of complications which can occur in your postmenopausal life, such as osteoporosis and cardiovascular problems, may require care from specialists based in other hospital departments.

## TREATMENTS

There is every chance that you will sail through your menopause without the need for any treatment. As we have seen, though, medical treatments can offer you relief from menopausal symptoms if these are proving troublesome, and if you are at risk of health problems like osteoporosis or cardiovascular disease, they can help to protect you against developing them. Most treatments are only taken for a few years, though if you do develop health problems in your postmenopausal life, these will probably require longer-term treatment.

### HRT: What is it?

The idea behind HRT is very simple. Menopausal symptoms and the increased risk of complications following the menopause are mostly due to the fact that oestrogen levels have fallen. HRT acts simply by replenishing the levels of this hormone. There are two basic forms of HRT.

1. **Oestrogen-only HRT** – this involves taking a small daily dose of oestrogen and is suitable for women who have had a hysterectomy and therefore no longer have a uterus.

2. **Combined HRT** – this is used for women who still have their uterus.

- *Combined sequential HRT* – involves taking small daily doses of oestrogen, plus a progestogen (a man-made, synthetic version of progesterone) for around 14 days in every 28. Sequential

combined HRT is designed to mimic the natural
menstrual cycle, and will cause monthly periods.
This is most suitable for women who are
perimenopausal, and so are still experiencing
some menstrual bleeding or for those within
12 months of their last period.

■ *Combined continuous HRT* – involves taking
small daily doses of oestrogen and progestogen
every day. This does not cause monthly periods
although it is usual to have irregular bleeding for
at least the first 3–6 months of therapy, after
which bleeding should stop completely.
Combined continuous HRT is not suitable for
women who are perimenopausal or for those
who have not yet been 12 months without a
menstrual period, but it used for women who
are clearly postmenopausal.

The drugs and medications referred to in this
Simple Guide are believed to be currently in
widespread use in the UK. Medical science can
evolve rapidly, but to the best of our knowledge, this
is a reasonable reflection of clinical practice at the
time of going to press.

Source: British National Formulary.

## PROGESTOGEN OR NO PROGESTOGEN?

You may be wondering why women with a uterus need to have progestogen added to their oestrogen HRT whereas women who have had a hysterectomy do not. This is because, on its own, oestrogen therapy can increase the risk of endometrial cancer (cancer of the endometrium, the lining of the uterus). If you have had a hysterectomy, there is of course no uterus to be affected (unless you have had endometriosis, in which case there may be sections of endometrial tissue remaining outside of the uterus). However, if you do still have your uterus, oestrogen-only therapy could put you at potential risk, but the added progestogen counteracts this effect of oestrogen on the endometrium.

### What different types of HRT are available?

HRT is available in a variety of different forms: a mixture of oestrogen-only medication, and those containing both oestrogen and progestogen. Although oestrogen tends to be referred to as a single hormone, the 'oestrogens' are in fact a whole group of individual hormones, including estradiol, estriol and estrone, each of which has similar effects. HRT containing oestrogens can contain one or a combination of more than one oestrogen.

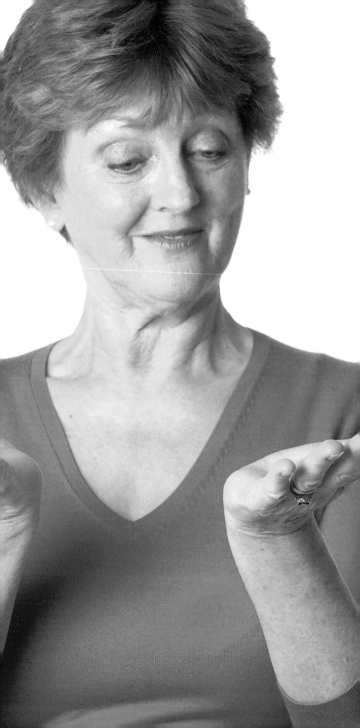

## THE FORMS OF HRT CURRENTLY AVAILABLE IN THE UK

| TABLETS | | |
|---|---|---|
| HRT type | Brand name | Tablets |
| Oestrogen only | Climaval® | * |
| | Elleste-Solo® | * |
| | FemTab® | * |
| | Hormonin® | * |
| | Ortho-Gynest® | * |
| | Ovestin® | * |
| | Premarin® | * |
| | Progynova® | * |
| | Vagifem® | * |
| | Zumenon® | * |
| Oestrogen + progestogen | Angeliq® | * |
| | Climagest® | * |
| | Climesse® | * |
| | Cyclo-Progynova® | * |
| | Elleste-Duet® | * |
| | Femapak® | * |
| | Femoston® | * |
| | FemTab® Sequi | * |
| | Indivina® | * |
| | Kliofem® | * |
| | Kliovance® | * |
| | Novofem® | * |
| | Nuvelle® | * |
| | Premique® | * |
| | Prempak-C® | * |
| | Tridestra® | * |
| | Trisequens® | * |
| Progestogen only* | Duphaston® HRT | * |
| | Micronor® HRT | * |
| | Provera® | * |

*The progestogens listed are designed to be used along with oestrogens to protect the endometrium and will not be prescribed on their own as HRT.

## PATCHES

| HRT type | Brand name | Patches |
|---|---|---|
| Oestrogen only | Elleste-Solo® MX | * |
| | Estraderm MX® | * |
| | Estraderm TTS® | * |
| | Estradot® | * |
| | Evorel® | * |
| | Fematrix® | * |
| | FemSeven® | * |
| | Progynova® TS | * |
| Oestrogen + progestogen | Estracombi® | * |
| | Evorel® | * |
| | Femapak® | * |
| | FemSeven® Conti | * |
| | FemSeven® Sequi | * |

## OTHER DEVICES

| HRT type | Brand name | Implants | Nasal spray | Vaginal ring | Gel | Vaginal cream | Pessary | Intra-uterine |
|---|---|---|---|---|---|---|---|---|
| Oestrogen only | Aerodiol® | | * | | | | | |
| | Estradiol implants | * | | | | | | |
| | Estring® | | | * | | | | |
| | Menoring® | | | * | | | | |
| | Oestrogel® | | | | * | | | |
| | Ortho-Gynest® | | | | | * | * | |
| | Ovestin® | | | | | * | | |
| | Premarin® | | | | | * | | |
| | Sandrena® | | | | * | | | |
| Progestogen only* | Mirena® | | | | | | | * |

*The progestogens listed are designed to be used along with oestrogens to protect the endometrium and will not be prescribed on their own as HRT.

### How is it taken?

HRT can be taken in a number of ways and depends on your personal preference, the reasons why you are taking it and your doctor's recommendation.

■ **Tablets**

Most commonly, HRT medication is available in tablet form. It is important that you follow your doctor's instructions very carefully with regards to when to take these tablets, particularly if you are taking combined sequential HRT, in which case the tablets you take will depend on how far through the 28-day cycle you are. Try to take your tablets at the same time each day, as this will help you to stick to a routine and avoid missing a dose.

■ **Patches**

HRT can be supplied as patches that you attach to your skin. Your doctor will advise you on where best to stick them, but make sure that they are not placed near your breasts or genitalia. Most patches are replaced after 3 or 4 days, although some can be left on for a whole week.

■ **Implants**

More rarely, oestrogen can be released slowly by a small cylindrical implant placed under your skin in your lower abdomen or buttock by a doctor. The implant will need to be replaced every 4–8 months or so, for as long as you need the treatment.

■ **Nasal spray**

If you are prescribed HRT in the form of a nasal spray, your doctor will ensure that you know exactly how to use it. Ask them what you should do if you find yourself suffering from a blocked nose – it is possible to apply the spray through the mouth but you will need to increase the dose in this case, and you should make sure that you know exactly what to do in this situation.

### ■ Vaginal ring

If you have your HRT in the form of a vaginal ring, this will be fitted into your vagina by a doctor or nurse. There are two different types of vaginal ring – one which releases oestrogen locally and therefore mainly targets local symptoms and one where the oestrogen is absorbed into your bloodstream, helping all symptoms. Your doctor will probably recommend that you keep the same ring for about 3 months before it needs replacing. You can learn to remove this when you have intercourse and replace it afterwards.

### ■ Gel

As in the case of patches, gels allow oestrogen to be absorbed through the skin into the body. Your doctor will advise you on where to apply the gel and how much to use. You must always apply the gel on unbroken, clean, dry skin, and must avoid applying it near to the breasts or genitalia. You should allow the applied gel to dry for about 5 minutes before covering the area of the skin with clothing. Make sure you wash your hands after using the gel and if the gel comes into contact with another person's skin (particularly if they are male), they must wash it off immediately.

■ **Vaginal cream or tablet**
This needs to be applied inside the vagina.
Although some creams come with applicators,
it is often easier to apply them by hand. Your
doctor will explain to you how you should use
the cream, how much of it to apply in one go
and how often you need to use it. It is
important to know that these creams may
damage latex condoms or diaphragms, so ask
your doctor for advice about contraception if
you are using vaginal creams.

■ **Pessary**
Similar to the vaginal ring, a pessary is a device
worn inside the vagina. You may be able to fit
it yourself or the doctor may suggest that they
do it for you. Initially, you may need to change
the pessary a few times a week, but this may
become less frequent with time.

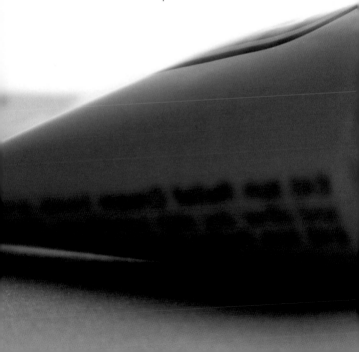

### ■ Intrauterine device

Available for the progestogen-only drug, Mirena®. A T-shaped plastic coil containing the progestogen is inserted into your uterus by a doctor. The fitting may be a little uncomfortable, and you may be offered a local anaesthetic. The intrauterine device will need to be changed after 5 years.

If you are unsure about any aspect of how to use your HRT, you should ask your doctor. If you need a quick answer to a question and your doctor is not available, a local pharmacist or the practice nurse will be able to give you the advice you need.

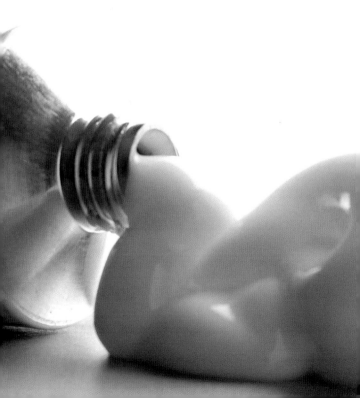

## What does it do?

■ Most of the symptoms associated with the menopause are at least partly due to the declining levels of oestrogen at this time. It is hardly surprising, then, that HRT is generally effective at reducing most of these symptoms. Vaginal creams, rings or tablets, in particular, are often chosen to relieve symptoms specifically affecting the genital region, such as vaginal dryness, though improvements can take several months. Other forms of HRT are often very effective at reducing the 'vasomotor' symptoms, such as hot flushes and sweating, usually within about 2–4 weeks.

■ Whether HRT can improve the psychological symptoms of menopause is less clear. The psychological impact of reaching the end of your reproductive life cannot really be altered with treatment, though if you are suffering from mood swings and feelings of anxiety or depression, these may be at least partly caused by your physical symptoms. Therefore, controlling these symptoms with HRT might indirectly improve your state of mental well-being.

■ As well as controlling menopausal symptoms, HRT can also help to ward off more long-term health problems. HRT is effective at reducing the risk of osteoporosis as it has a protective effect on bone density. Although this effect is beneficial, oestrogen is not now recommended for the express purpose of preserving bone strength, primarily because of safety concerns associated with its long-term use. There is also some evidence that HRT can reduce your risk of colorectal cancer.

■ Although HRT was previously thought to delay or reduce the risk of Alzheimer's disease, and to preserve memory, this has not been borne out by long-term clinical trials like the Women's Health Initiative memory study, which showed that taking HRT after the age of 65 actually increased the risk of developing dementia.

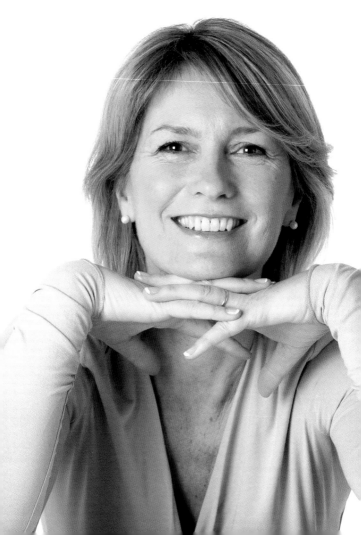

### Is it safe?

HRT might not cause many immediately apparent side-effects, and may appear to be the obvious solution to make the menopausal transition easier, but unfortunately some serious safety issues have been recognised in recent years that we need to consider. These relate to the potential of HRT to slightly increase the risk of a number of serious health problems.

There has been a lot of media coverage of the health risks associated with HRT, prompting many women to seek alternative treatment options. Remember, though, that you are not being left to make a decision on your own as to whether you think HRT is safe for you.

The Committee on Safety of Medicines (CSM) is an independent advisory committee which advises government health ministers on which medicines are safe and effective for people to use. The CSM has released a number of reports and press releases over the last few years, documenting their findings on the effects of HRT on the risk of health problems such as heart disease, stroke, dementia, breast cancer, endometrial cancer and ovarian cancer. Much of this guidance has been developed on the basis of results from two major studies which included women taking HRT.

- The **Women's Health Initiative (WHI)** was designed in the early 1990s to be a strictly controlled scientific study into various strategies which might improve health and life expectancy amongst women between the ages of 50 and 79. Women were given a placebo (inactive drug) or HRT (oestrogen only if the woman had had a hysterectomy or combined oestrogen plus progesterone if not).

- The **Million Women Study (MWS)** was not so much a controlled scientific trial, but an 'observational' study of over 1 million women (aged 50–64) attending the NHS Breast Screening Programme in the UK. Although this study looked at huge numbers of women, some experts have cast doubt over the way that the data have been collected and interpreted.

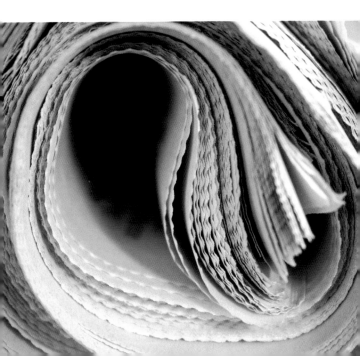

The general consensus arising from these studies, as outlined in the British Menopause Society Council Consensus Statement on Hormone Replacement Therapy (*www.the-bms.org/consensus.htm*), is that HRT has the potential to offer more benefit than harm, providing that the appropriate dose, form of administration (e.g. tablet, cream) and combination of hormones is used. It is up to you and your doctor to establish the lowest dose of HRT that is effective for you, and to ensure that the benefits you get from the drugs outweigh the risks. In contrast, the CSM does not recommend HRT, except for the short-term relief of menopausal symptoms.

These studies have made it clear, however, that, except in rare cases, it is not reasonable to use HRT as a means of preventing long-term diseases. Indefinite use of HRT might reduce your risk of osteoporosis, but may increase your risk of breast cancer and cardiovascular problems at the same time. The combined HRT part of the WHI study was actually stopped earlier than planned, when most women had received just over 5 years of oestrogen and progestogen treatment, because the risk of breast cancer, in particular, was climbing too high.

In short, then, HRT is suitable for the relief of menopausal symptoms for up to 5 years, unless your doctor considers it too risky on the basis of your own medical situation (e.g. history of deep vein thrombosis or suspected breast cancer). Your doctor will provide the risk and benefit information which you will need to carefully consider in order to make a decision about

whether you wish to take HRT for longer than
5 years of continuous treatment. You do not have
to make this choice alone. Talk it over with your
doctor and make sure you arrive at a decision that
you are happy with. If you have a premature
menopause, your doctor may suggest that you take
HRT up until the age of the average menopause
(we will look at this in more detail later).

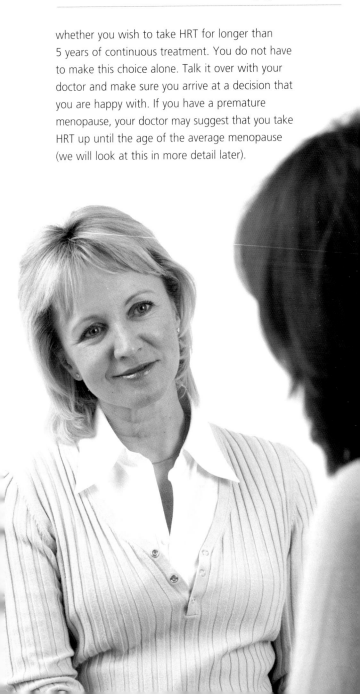

## Relative and absolute risks

The studies of HRT safety have sparked a lot of press coverage in the last few years, and the way that the media have reported the findings has created widespread mistrust of the drugs. The WHI study, in particular, has been the subject of much attention. However, it is important to be aware that the media have concentrated quite heavily on one aspect of the data from the WHI, known as the *relative risks*. Relative risks are used to compare the risk of an event in two groups of people.

The trouble with using relative risks on their own is that it is quite easy to lose sight of the real meaning of the numbers. Imagine a clinical trial where people taking a drug were found to be twice as likely to get a particular disease as people who had taken a placebo instead. You might be concerned that the drug was dangerous. However, if you also knew that that disease was incredibly rare – say only one-in-a-million people normally get it in their lifetime, increased to two-in-a-million if taking the drug – you might consider that it was well worth taking that risk, given the benefits that the drug could offer you. *Absolute risk* data, which were also calculated during the WHI study, tell us the chance that a person will develop a disease in a particular time period, and this helps to keep the relative risk data in perspective.

Let's look at the actual data from the WHI study. The relative risk of developing breast cancer when taking combined oestrogen and progestogen HRT compared with placebo was 1.26. This means that for every one woman who developed breast cancer after taking placebo, 1.26 women would be expected to develop the disease after taking combined HRT for about 5 years. (Obviously you cannot have fractions of women – these are just statistics to help to illustrate the size of the effect!) Whilst this relative risk might at initial glance seem quite alarming, the absolute risk (which was less frequently reported by the media) revealed that this translates to an extra eight women out of every 10,000 developing breast cancer in a year. This is clearly an increased risk, but perhaps one that some women would be prepared to consider taking.

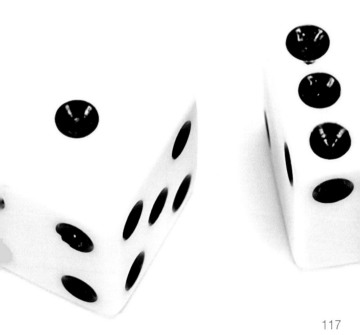

**KEY DATA FROM THE WHI STUDY AFTER 5 YEARS OF
TREATMENT WITH COMBINED HRT**

| Condition |
| --- |
| Breast cancer |
| Coronary heart disease |
| Stroke |
| Pulmonary embolism (a blood clot in the vessels carrying blood to the lungs) |
| Colorectal cancer (cancer of the large bowel or rectum) |
| Hip fracture |

### Stopping HRT

When it comes to stopping your HRT treatment, depending on the dose you are taking, your doctor may decide that it is best to gradually reduce the dose rather than to stop it abruptly. This can help to minimise the risk of you suffering symptoms again. You may find that menopausal symptoms come back for a while after stopping HRT treatment, but then resolve on their own.

If you have any concerns – for example, if you are worried that you might have been on HRT for too long – do not be tempted to stop your HRT without first consulting your doctor.

| Relative risk | Absolute risk (change in number of cases per 10,000 women per year) |
|---|---|
| 1.26 | 8 more |
| 1.29 | 7 more |
| 1.41 | 8 more |
| | |
| 2.13 | 8 more |
| 0.63 | 6 fewer |
| 0.66 | 5 fewer |

## OTHER HORMONE-BASED TREATMENTS

### Tibolone

Tibolone is regarded as a form of HRT. In contrast to more conventional HRT, however, in which the hormones oestrogen and progesterone are taken separately, tibolone is a single man-made (synthetic) product which mimics oestrogen and progesterone, as well as showing some testosterone-like activity too. It is similar, therefore, to combined continuous HRT. It offers similar benefits, though it appears to be more effective than conventional HRT in improving women's sex drive – probably by virtue of its testosterone-like activity (see overleaf). Tibolone is also subject to the same safety concerns as conventional HRT, and so your doctor will carefully consider your dose and duration of treatment, keeping both to a minimum. Tibolone (brand name Livial®), is only available in tablet form, and these are taken daily.

### Testosterone

Testosterone is generally thought of as a male hormone, but a woman's ovaries and adrenal glands (a pair of glands located above the kidneys) produce some too. Levels of testosterone will therefore drop around the time of the menopause, and this is thought to contribute to the loss of libido suffered by some women. There is some evidence that testosterone treatment can offer some improvement to a woman's sex drive around the time of her menopause and perhaps reduce hot flushes. Testosterone also appears to exaggerate the effects of the oestrogen in HRT, though it is not clear why this happens.

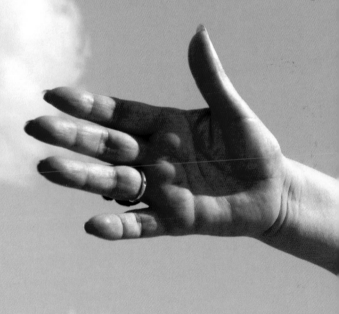

It is still quite rare for women to be prescribed testosterone. However, if your doctor thinks that you would benefit from testosterone therapy in addition to conventional HRT, they will offer you an implant which will need to be replaced every 4–8 months. There is a concern that testosterone treatment could cause women to show signs of certain masculine features, such as facial hair and a deeper voice. However, this does not usually happen with the low doses of testosterone used to treat women. Testosterone has not yet been used in women for long enough to be certain about potential long-term health risks.

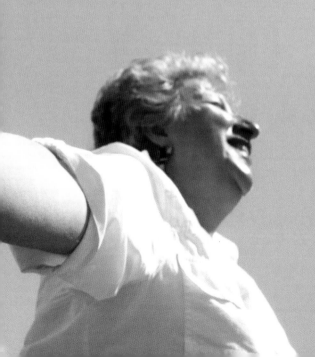

## OTHER TREATMENTS FOR VASOMOTOR SYMPTOMS

### Clonidine

This drug is more commonly used to treat high blood pressure and migraine, but it appears to have some benefits in reducing hot flushes. It is thought to do this by stabilising blood vessel calibre, and therefore improving temperature regulation in the body (see *Simple science* page 58). Clonidine (Catapres® and Dixarit®), available in tablet form may cause unpleasant side-effects including a dry mouth and drowsiness. Your doctor may prescribe it to prevent your hot flushes instead of HRT.

### Selective serotonin reuptake inhibitors

Selective serotonin reuptake inhibitors (SSRIs) are a class of drugs normally used to treat depression, but as we saw in *Simple science* (page 60), they also appear to reduce hot flushes. This has not yet been tested fully in large scale clinical trials, and these drugs are not licensed for use as a treatment for menopausal vasomotor symptoms. However, as in the case of the effects of HRT on bone, the potential improvement to hot flushes can be seen as a kind of helpful side-effect of these antidepressant drugs.

## OFF-LICENCE INDICATIONS

Before they can be used in people, all drugs must be granted a licence by the Medicines and Healthcare products Regulatory Agency (MHRA). The licence will set out exactly which diseases and conditions the drug can legally be used to treat. Any medicinal use of the drug that is not covered in the terms of the licence is called an 'off-licence indication'. Your doctor may prescribe you a drug for an off-licence indication, such as the use of an SSRI for relief of hot flushes, but this is done at their discretion.

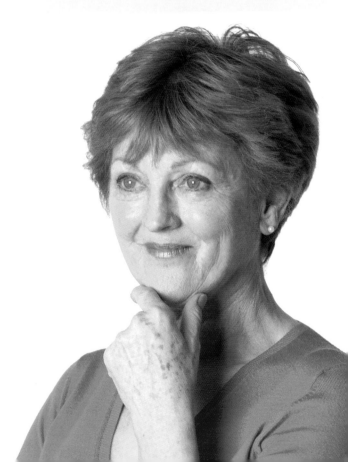

## COMPLEMENTARY AND ALTERNATIVE THERAPIES

Complementary and alternative medicine (i.e. treatment not involving conventional drugs or surgery) has been gaining popularity in recent years. Given the (sometimes exaggerated) risks that can be associated with HRT, women have become increasingly keen to search for complementary therapies that they can use for menopausal symptoms. There is very little formal evidence that these treatments are effective in this respect, but this is not to say that they cannot benefit you.

Complementary and alternative medicine is also gaining support from doctors in the UK, and many will be happy to advise you on which treatments may be of benefit to you. Even if you do not want to take any prescription medications for your menopausal symptoms, it is important to seek your doctor's advice when considering whether to try a complementary medicine option. Complementary medicines are not subject to the same strict safety tests that other drugs have to go through. Just because a dietary supplement, for example, comes from a natural source, this does not mean it is safe, and some complementary health products have the potential to affect the way that other drugs work in your body.

Complementary and alternative medicine for menopausal symptoms is largely focused on herbalism. There are a number of herbal remedies that have been used in treating menopausal symptoms. Claims about their effectiveness and safety generally relate to experience rather than controlled scientific studies, though these are increasingly being carried out. The most common herbal remedies include:

- black cohosh
- agnus castus (monk's pepper/chasteberry extract)
- evening primrose oil
- gingko biloba
- dong quai
- ginseng
- sage
- St John's wort.

Other complementary and alternative treatments include:

- homeopathy
- reflexology
- hypnosis
- acupuncture
- aromatherapy
- yoga.

## TREATMENTS FOR HEAVY BLEEDING

As we have seen, prior to the menopause, your menstrual periods can become quite changeable, both in their frequency and in how heavy they are. Many women suffer with particularly heavy periods (menorrhagia) for some time before they stop menstruating altogether. There are a number of treatments that can help to control this uncomfortable and constraining problem:

■ non-steroidal anti-inflammatory drugs (NSAIDs) to reduce pain (e.g. ibuprofen)

■ drugs which reduce bleeding (tranexamic acid [Cyklokapron®] and etamsylate [Dicynene®])

■ progestogen-only therapy to reduce the amount of uterus lining present and therefore available to be shed during each period (Mirena®, intrauterine system [IUS])

■ surgery (hysterectomy or endometrial ablation, which destroys the lining of the uterus).

## TREATMENT OF PSYCHOLOGICAL SYMPTOMS

If you are finding the psychological impact of the menopause very difficult, your doctor can suggest a range of options. HRT itself is unlikely to help a great deal with the emotional side of things. However, counselling – either one-to-one or in a group – with a trained professional can really help you to come to terms with the changes that are happening in your life. Your GP will be able to put you in touch with a counsellor.

If you do not find counselling very helpful, or if your doctor thinks that your symptoms warrant it, he or she may prescribe you antidepressant tablets. These can have side-effects, but some of these can be beneficial, as we have seen (e.g. improving hot flushes). You may not need to take antidepressant medication for very long, but remember that it will take 10–14 days to get any benefit and a good few weeks to take full effect, and that it can cause side-effects to stop taking it suddenly. Always make sure you follow your doctor's instructions carefully.

Of course, it is always important to turn to your friends and family for support. Remember, though, that it may be distressing for your loved ones to see you behaving out of character, so try to be understanding if they seem confused or upset themselves. Maintaining an active social life will help you to overcome feelings of emotional difficulty. Try not to let your physical symptoms prevent you from doing this.

**For more information see**
**Depression**

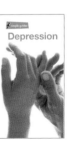

## TREATMENT OF UROGENITAL SYMPTOMS

As we have seen, HRT can help to improve vaginal dryness, particularly when applied as a cream or vaginal tablet to the genital area. Vaginal lubricants or moisturisers may, however, offer a more direct solution to the problem of vaginal dryness. Water-soluble lubricants, such as KY Jelly® or Replens®, are available from your pharmacist. KY jelly, if applied before sexual intercourse, can help relieve dryness temporarily and make intercourse more comfortable. Replens, if used regularly for a few days, is retained in the vaginal walls, making them more moist for a length of time.

HRT may also offer some relief from incontinence. However, incontinence may turn out to be a more long-term problem than some other menopausal symptoms, and you cannot take HRT indefinitely. Other strategies for treating incontinence include:

- pelvic floor exercises

- vaginal cones (plastic weights that you hold in your vagina for about 15 minutes – a way to make pelvic floor exercises easier to do)

- electrical stimulation (to exercise your pelvic floor muscles for you)

- collagen implants

- drug treatments (e.g. duloxetine [Yentreve®], tolterodine [Detrusitol®]).

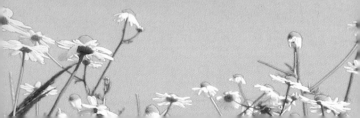

## DEALING WITH PREMATURE MENOPAUSE

If you think that your menopause is coming or has come too early, it is important that you see your doctor, even if you feel fine and are able to cope. From the point of view of your future health, having your menopause early puts you at increased risk of osteoporosis and other postmenopausal complications compared with a woman who has her menopause in her late 40s or early 50s. This is because you spend more of your life in the absence of the protective effects of oestrogen. For this reason, your doctor may suggest that you take HRT up until the average age of menopause (51 years).

A major issue for some women who have their menopause is that of infertility. If the menopause arrives during your thirties, or even earlier, there is a chance that you may have still been intending to have children. If you still have your uterus intact, one option you may wish to speak to your doctor about is IVF (*in vitro* fertilisation). This involves eggs from a donor being fertilised by your partner's sperm in a laboratory. The embryos that hopefully result from this are then implanted into your uterus, and the baby develops there naturally.

For more information on coping with premature menopause, see *www.daisynetwork.org.uk*

## THE LONG AND SHORT OF IT

So should you be worried about the menopause? No, you needn't worry about it. You may be lucky, and not be troubled by symptoms for the few years surrounding your menopause. If you have led a healthy, active lifestyle and do not have any family history of serious health problems, the chances are that the menopause can be an entirely positive transition in your life. It will free you of menstrual periods and the need for contraception, and give you a good incentive to maintain your healthy lifestyle and diet.

Even if you do suffer distressing symptoms, there are a range of treatments available to relieve them, and you can rest safe in the knowledge that most of them should completely resolve within a few years anyway. Some problems, particularly those relating to genital problems, can worsen with time, and you may therefore need ongoing treatment.

It is important to be aware of the implications of your declining oestrogen levels. If you understand the reasons why your bones may weaken and your cardiovascular system is at more risk after the menopause, you will be more aware of the importance of protecting them. Make sure that your doctor explains to you what you can do to minimise your risk of developing serious health problems after the menopause, and know the signs to look out for that will tell you that something is not right.

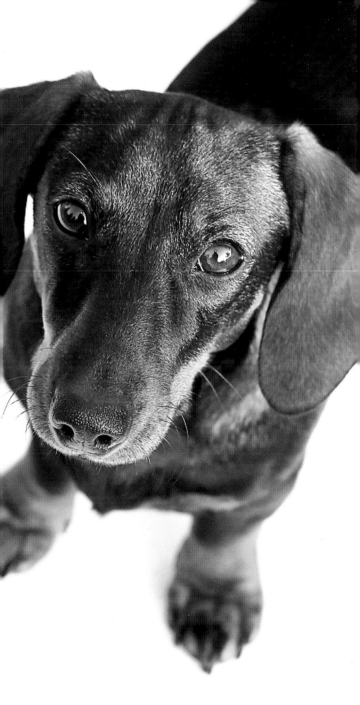

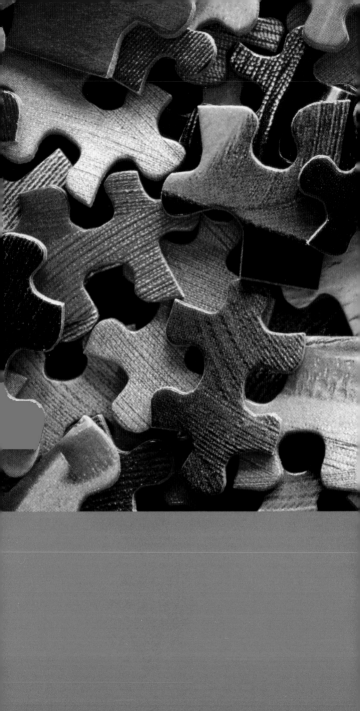

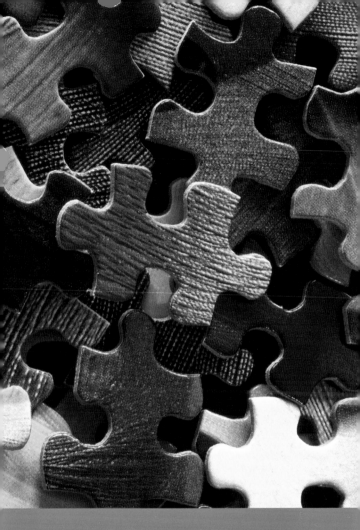

# Simple
# extras

## FURTHER READING

- **Osteoporosis (Simple Guide)**
  CSF Medical Communications Ltd, 2006
  ISBN: 1-905466-11-0, £5.99
  *www.bestmedicine.com*

- **Arthritis (Simple Guide)**
  CSF Medical Communications Ltd, 2006
  ISBN: 1-905466-12-9, £5.99
  *www.bestmedicine.com*

- **Blood Pressure (Simple Guide)**
  CSF Medical Communications Ltd, 2005
  ISBN: 1-905466-04-8, £5.99
  *www.bestmedicine.com*

- **Cholesterol (Simple Guide)**
  CSF Medical Communications Ltd, 2005
  ISBN: 1-905466-05-6, £5.99
  *www.bestmedicine.com*

- **Type 2 Diabetes (Simple Guide)**
  CSF Medical Communications Ltd, 2005
  ISBN: 1-905466-02-1, £5.99
  *www.bestmedicine.com*

- **Depression (Simple Guide)**
  CSF Medical Communications Ltd, 2005
  ISBN: 1-905466-03-X, £5.99
  *www.bestmedicine.com*

- *www.the-bms.org/consensus.htm*
  (British Menopause Society Council Consensus
  Statement on Hormone Replacement Therapy)

- *www.mhra.gov.uk/home/groups/pl-p/
  documents/drugsafetymessage/con019453.pdf*
  (Committee of Safety of Medicine statement on
  safety of HRT)

- *www.menopausematters.co.uk*

- *www.food.gov.uk*

## USEFUL CONTACTS

**British Menopause Society**
4–6 Eton Place
Marlow
Buckinghamshire
SL7 2QA
Tel: 01628 890199
Fax: 01628 474042
Website: *www.the-bms.org*

**The Daisy Network**
(Premature Menopause Support Group)
PO Box 183
Rossendale
BB4 6WZ
Website: *www.daisynetwork.org.uk*

**The Hysterectomy Association**
60 Redwood House
Charlton Down
Dorchester
Dorset
DT2 9UH
Tel: 0871 7811141
Website: *www.hysterectomy-association.org.uk*

**National Osteoporosis Society**
Camerton
Bath
BA2 0PJ
Osteoporosis helpline: 0845 4500230
General telephone enquiries: 01761 471771
Website: *www.nos.org.uk*

■ **NHS Direct**
NHS Direct Line: 0845 46 47
Website: *www.nhsdirect.nhs.uk*

■ **The British Complementary Medicine Association**
PO Box 2074
Seaford BN25 1HQ
Tel: 0845 345 5977
Email: *info@bcma.co.uk*
Website: *www.bcma.co.uk*

■ **The Patients Association**
The Patients Association is a UK charity which represents patient rights, influences health policy and campaigns for better patient care.
**Contact details:**
PO Box 935
Harrow
Middlesex
HA1 3YJ
Helpline: 0845 6084455
Email: *mailbox@patients-association.com*
Website: *www.patients-association.com*

## SIMPLE GUIDE QUESTIONNAIRE

Dear reader,

We would love to know what you thought of this Simple Guide. Please take a few moments to fill out this short questionnaire and return it to us at the FREEPOST address below.

**CSF Medical Communications Ltd**
FREEPOST NAT5703
Witney
OX29 8BR

### SO WHAT DID YOU THINK?

**Which Simple Guide have you just read?**

_____

**Where did you buy it (store/town)?**

_____

**Who did you buy it for?**

☐ Myself      ☐ Friend      ☐ Relative
☐ Patient     ☐ Other

**Where did you hear about the Simple Guides?**

☐ They were recommended to me      ☐ Internet
☐ Stumbled across them              ☐ Other

**Did it meet with your expectations?**

☐ Exceeded      ☐ Met all
☐ Met most      ☐ Fell below

**Was there anything you particularly liked?**

_____

_____

_____

**Was there anything we could have improved?**

_____

_____

_____

**WHO ARE YOU?**

Name: _____

Address: _____

_____

_____

Tel: _____

Email: _____

**How old are you?**

☐ Under 25    ☐ 25–34    ☐ 35–44
☐ 45–54       ☐ 55–64    ☐ 65+

**Are you...**    ☐ Male    ☐ Female

**Do you suffer from a long-term medical condition? If so, please specify.**

_____

**WHAT NEXT?**

**What other topics would you like to see covered in future Simple Guides?**

Thanks,
        the Simple Guides team